"People are born resourceful and they become skillful and 'thoughtful' when they genuinely care about what they are doing."

- Frank R. Wilson, *The Hand*

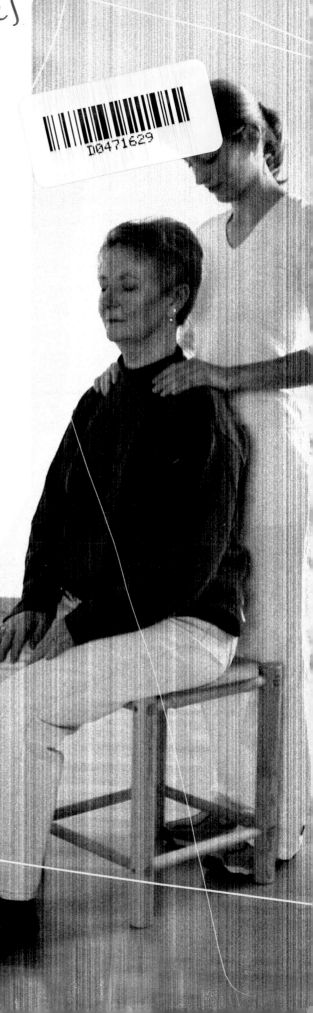

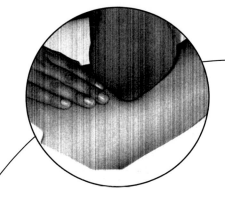

Body Mechanics for Manual Therapists

A Functional Approach to Self-Care

Barbara Frye, LMP, GCFP
Licensed Massage Practitioner
Guild Certified Feldenkrais Practitioner[CM]

Published by
Fryetag Publishing
P.O. Box 2688
Stanwood, WA 98292
Toll Free: (877) 474-1001

ISBN 0-9700521-1-1

Edited by
Kathleen Domeisen

REVIEWERS

Clint Chandler, LMP, CNMT
Senior Faculty, Boulder College of Massage Therapy
Jerome Perlinski National Teacher of the Year, 2002
Boulder, Colorado

Tim Herbert
National Sales Director, CustomCraftworks
Eugene, Oregon

Dr. Joseph E. Muscolino, DC
Faculty, Connecticut Center for Massage Therapy
Author of *The Muscular System Manual &*
The Musculoskeletal Anatomy Coloring Book
Redding, Connecticut

Diana L. Thompson, LMP
Author of *Hands Heal: Communication, Documentation, and Insurance Billing*
for Manual Therapists
Seattle, Washington

Graphic design and production by
Jackie Phillips

Illustration by Jackie Phillips
Figure 4.9a, 4.9b, 6.3

Illustration by Robin Dorn
Figure 5.4, 5.5, 5.6, 5.7, 5.8, 5.22, 6.5, 7.16, 9.18, Appendix D Stretches

Printed by
Cenveo
Seattle, WA

 Printed on recycled paper.

DISCLAIMER
The publisher is not responsible for any injury resulting from any material contained
herein. The purpose of this book is to provide information for manual therapists on
the subject of body mechanics. This book does not offer medical advice to the reader and is not intended as a replacement for appropriate health care and treatment.
For such advice, readers should consult a licensed physician.

Table of Contents

Foreward

Massage therapy is a very powerful healing tool for the body, mind, heart and soul. Indeed, educated touch that is mindful and comes from the heart can be transformational. When people make the decision to begin massage therapy school, this is likely the main reason that motivates them to enter the field; they desire to help and heal people through the gift of touch. I am sure that if you were to speak to these new students of massage and have them describe a session in which a therapist is massaging a client, they would likely focus on all the healing benefits of massage for the client. If they do think of the session from the point of view of the therapist, it would probably be to describe the mindful and heartfelt intention of the therapist to heal the client. In effect, they are still viewing the massage session from the perspective of the client and his/her healing process. All this is natural and noble. In fact, it is this desire on the part of massage therapists to help other people through their touch that makes the field of massage such a wonderful and successful field.

However, what I believe most aspiring massage therapists do not fully realize is that the process of giving a massage and the process of receiving a massage can be quite different. Even if the therapist and client share a mindful and heartfelt connection, it is the client that receives the physical benefits of the massage, whereas it is the therapist who must work on a physical level to deliver the massage. Indeed, the physical process of giving a massage can be hard work for the body of the therapist!

This hard work may not be apparent at first. When only a few massages need to be given, whether we work in an efficient manner or not, we can usually get away with giving massages to our fellow students or to our clients when we first enter the field. But as massage after massage is done, the physical demands on the part of the therapist can add up, resulting in fatigue and eventually injury. This is especially true if the therapist does not have good body mechanics when giving massage! Unfortunately, in the place of good body mechanics, many therapists work inefficiently and excessively tax the muscles of their body. They achieve the result of giving the massage by working the muscles of their body much harder than they need to. In effect, instead of being efficient and graceful with their body mechanics, they 'muscle' the massage. However, this method can last only so long before problems develop. Even large, strong, powerful individuals will eventually find out that 'muscling' a massage does not work and they too will fatigue and develop injuries. Unfortunately, once the massage therapist is in pain, it is hard to deliver a mindful and heartfelt massage to the client because all that the therapist can feel is the pain in his/her own body.

This is where Barbara Frye's book, *Body Mechanics for Manual Therapists,* is so valuable. In the same manner that people study proper posture and the use of body mechanics in the workplace for other professions, i.e., the study of 'ergonomics', Barbara Frye applies these same ergonomic principles to the field of massage therapy. There are ten chapters that cover everything from the basic principles of good body mechanics, to the specific application of these proper body mechanics to each position in which a massage therapist might work, e.g., standing, sitting, bending etc. Further, Barbara discusses the application of proper body mechanics to such topics as applying pressure, and pushing and pulling strokes. There is even an appendix that addresses the application of massage to working on surfaces other than a massage table (for example, chair massage or the floor for shiatsu), proper mechanics for massage therapists working in a spa environment, and stretching and troubleshooting injuries common to manual therapists.

All of this is placed into a book that is easy to read because it is written in a simple and straight-forward manner, with humor interjected along the way. The illustrations are also simple and clear, enabling the reader to easily visualize the proper body mechanics that are being described in the text. Further, this book is written in an interactive fashion giving the reader a lot of space for exploration and thought, and perhaps even more importantly, allowing its use as a workbook in the classroom at a massage school. For those schools that choose to adopt this book as a textbook in their curriculum, there is also a companion teachers' manual that is available.

I recommend that proper body mechanics be taught at every massage and bodywork school. Further, I recommend that this subject be taught at the very inception of the students' study, before bad habits are learned and patterned. Just as we in the health field instruct our clients on what the proper postures and uses of our body are, massage therapists need to follow the same principles as they carry on their work. Barbara Frye's book helps therapists do that, and helps massage therapy schools teach these principles to their students; and it accomplishes this in an easy and entertaining manner!

So, to increase the longevity of your practice and prevent physical burnout, and in turn enable you to comfortably deliver a better and more healthful massage to your clients now and into the future, I heartily recommend *Body Mechanics for Manual Therapists* to you.

Dr. Joseph E. Muscolino
Redding, Connecticut

Preface

Over the years, my experience as an educator has taught me that in order to assist students to learn a subject successfully, kinesthetic, cognitive and environmental elements must be present in the learning process. Creativity and playfulness, in my opinion, must also be woven in. With this philosophy in mind, I have written the second edition of *Body Mechanics for Manual Therapists,* as an in-class, hands-on study guide for all students of bodywork, and as a reference for practicing manual therapists. This text integrates all of the above-mentioned elements with the intention of leading you, the reader, toward an enjoyable and successful development of a self-care strategy. I would like to share with you how this edition goes about accomplishing this goal:

Cognitive learning gives you the opportunity to think about each concept. This begins with the clearly and concisely written explanations. In every chapter, you also have the opportunity to think about and write responses to provocative questions asked in the section called *Something to think about.* An element that also adds to the cognitive learning process is *Consider this.* It offers quotes and facts that give insight, including the knowledge and expertise of Dr. Joseph Muscolino, DC, author of *The Muscular System Manual.*

Kinesthetic learning is incorporated into the *Self-observation* and/or *Partner practice* lessons. These exercises assist you to physically experience each of the major concepts covered in every chapter. Through your kinesthetic experiences, you sense how specific movements influence particular functions of your body mechanics, for example, sensing how bending from your hip joints can produce positive results when lifting your client's leg. These kinesthetic experiences lead you to the discovery of effective and successful body mechanics.

Environmental learning is crucial so that you understand how the material relates to the world around you. Therefore, every chapter has *Practice tips* and *Client education tips,* giving you ideas on how to integrate the material into your everyday practice as a manual therapist.

I have chosen to integrate the important elements of **creativity and playfulness**, primarily, into the visual aspect of the text. Adding these elements allowed me the opportunity to turn an otherwise "dry" and somewhat complex subject into one that is easy and fun to understand and experience. As you read this book, I want each page to stimulate your learning experience in a positive and exciting way.

There are also some new additions I would like to tell you about: The first edition included a chapter called *The Basics.* In this edition,

---

When working through the Self-observation and Partner practice lessons, keep a few things in mind:

Take your time and go through each lesson slowly. You can always go back and review them at a faster pace. You will learn much faster if you, at first, move slowly and with awareness.

Always rest when you need to. There are plenty of rest breaks written into each lesson, but if you need to rest before they come up, please feel free to do so.

Be playful. If a movement feels strange or unfamiliar to you, don't take it too seriously and/or feel that you are doing something wrong. Just notice how it feels and move on. You can re-visit any exercise or movement at a later time. Every lesson has been specifically written so that you have the opportunity to feel and sense a variety of movement choices.

Before beginning a Partner practice, let your partner know what you will be asking of him or her. Give a general idea of the lesson and make sure that your partner feels comfortable with what you will be doing together. Whenever possible, practice with a variety of body types; clients come in all shapes and sizes.

And finally, allow yourself to discover what movements and body mechanics feel most effective for you. This text will guide you toward an effective use of your body, but you are the only person who can make the final choice of what feels right for you.

it has been expanded into two chapters called *Outside basics* and *Inside basics*. New information in these chapters include **table and chair consumer tips**, **breathing** and **hydration**. An enhanced *Tools of the trade* chapter includes **use of the foot and lower leg** for implementing massage. You will find new appendices including information on how to apply the concepts learned to **spa therapy** and **transferring clients**. An appendix called **Troubleshooting common repetitive injuries** has also been added.

Whether you are a student or a therapist in practice, I wish you an enjoyable and successful experience as you read and work your way through *Body Mechanics for Manual Therapists*.

Warm Regards,
Barbara Frye, LMP, GCFP

Acknowledgments

From the Swiss Alps, to the Seattle Cascades, to a little island called Maui, there have been many people who, in one way or the other, have supported this process. A big thank you and hug to:

Jackie Phillips, for giving life to each page of this book - your talents never cease to amaze me. I hope you are as delighted with the results as I am. It has been an absolute pleasure and honor working with you —I have enjoyed every moment. Du bist wirklich eine Superfrau!

Kathleen Domeisen, my American anchor in der Schweiz, for reading and reading and reading again. Our ongoing comma discussions still keep me awake at night. I will always remember that a Panda eats, shoots and leaves!

Christina Bachmann, Karin Dittli, Kathleen Domeisen, Iris Fritschi, Enid Frye, Denise Heinzmann, Marc Heinzmann, Regula Lienert, Angela Nacke, Phillip Penner, Claudia Rechsteiner, and Claudia Roos fuer eure Geduld und eure Unterstuetzung beim Photografieren.

My Fryetag publishing team, none of this would be possible without you, especially now that we know that I totally suck when it comes to wrapping! I love you both muchly!

Diana Thompson, for continuing to lead the way. Auf Wiedersehen!

Joe Muscolino, for barely knowing me, but agreeing to be a part of this project. Your expertise, feedback and even our friendly disagreements have made this a better book.

Robin Dorn, for your permission to use some "old friends" from the first edition.

CustomCraftworks, especially Tim Herbert, for your enthusiasm, promotion and commitment to self-care education.

Kate Bromley, Marissa Brooks, Paula Pelletier Butler, Leslie Grounds, Yvonne La Seur, Coleen Renee, Marty Ryan and Ann Wardell, for your initial feedback and suggestions - they have been integrated into this edition.

Drew Biel, Greg Bolton, Pete Darcey, Angel DiBenedetto, Barb Ford, Robert Land, Gayle MacDonald, Brenda Muscatell, Jeff Thompson, Michael Thurnherr and Charlotte Versagi for your help, promotion, good advice, expertise and generous spirit.

The instructors, students and manual therapists who used the first edition and gave feedback. Because of you, this edition is more complete.

Clint Chandler, for your continued support.

Jerry Karzen and Jeff Haller, for your understanding of and dedication to the fundamental teachings of Moshe Feldenkrais. You have both inspired and driven me to be a better practitioner.

Angela Nacke, for your constant encouragement and willingness to have conversations, no matter the time of day. You have shown me that writing a book doesn't have to be so difficult. Big love.

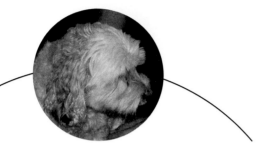

In memory of Wasabi

Whenever I say your name
Let there be no mistake
that day will last forever

Sting
Whenever I Say Your Name

1 Awareness is the Key

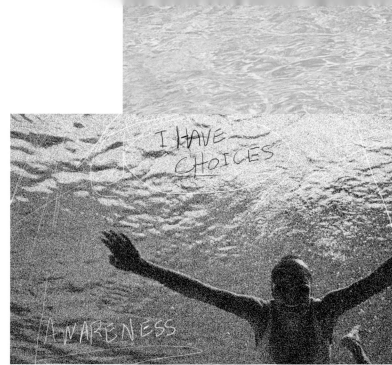

Introduction

There is no time like the present to develop self-care, prevent injury and foster good health. The recent study showing that 78% of massage professionals have experienced a work-related injury is a compelling reason to begin this process.[1] There is, however, no quick and easy way to develop self-care. The process of learning how to maintain your health and the longevity of your practice is an ongoing one and must be fostered in your own personal way.

This chapter will begin the process of developing a self-care strategy, and lays the foundation for the book. You will learn why self-care begins with developing body awareness and how, once you become aware of your body, you can begin to identify your movement habits. You will discover that as you become aware of your body and habits of movement, you can begin to discover which movement habits serve you and which ones hinder and cause you discomfort. Finally, you will learn that developing body awareness, by identifying your movement habits and sensing the difference between ease and effort, leads to an awareness of choice. Having choices gives you the opportunity to develop a wide range of effective body mechanics, ultimately yielding a sound and effective self-care strategy and a longevity of practice.

Before you read this chapter…

How would you rate your body awareness on an everyday basis?

always aware   mostly aware   sometimes aware   not very aware

What part of your body are you most aware of?
- upper body
- lower body
- head
- other_____

What part of your body are you least aware of?
- upper body
- lower body
- rib cage
- other_____

Describe 5 of your daily habits. e.g., brushing your teeth after eating.
1. _____
2. _____
3. _____
4. _____
5. _____

Describe an everyday activity that you feel is easy and pleasurable.
_____
_____

Describe an everyday activity that you feel is difficult and uncomfortable.
_____
_____

How aware are you of the choices you have?
- always
- mostly
- sometimes
- never

Body awareness

Before we can discuss the specifics concerning your body mechanics, we must first discuss your body awareness. Body awareness is where developing a sound self-care strategy and effective body mechanics all begins. Without it, we go blindly through our work, not realizing how our movements, responses, sensations and feelings affect our health.

Body awareness can be defined as a mindfulness of your body's movements, responses, sensations and feelings. As you develop this mindfulness, you become more aware of subtle movement patterns, such as, the posture of your head when you work or the shifting of your weight when you stand. Developing body awareness requires you to become more self-observant, not only when you are performing manual therapy, but also during your everyday life.

Incorporating a few minutes of self-observation into your sessions is an easy and pro-active way to develop body awareness. Over time, you will discover that attaining body awareness provides you with more information about yourself and how you work. This insightful attentiveness will help you make healthy choices between body mechanics that precede occupational injury and body mechanics that prevent occupational injury.

At this point, your level of body awareness may be well-developed or you may be just starting to discover it. Whatever your level of awareness, gaining more will provide you with the invaluable information needed to continue to foster your self-care, prevent injury and become more self-reliant.

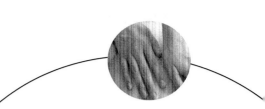

Practice tip 1.1

Include a few moments of self-observation in your workday. For example, observe how you are breathing at a particular moment. You don't need to observe several things, just one or two is fine. Make it interesting for yourself so that you continue to do it each day.

Something to think about...

When you think of "body awareness", what comes to mind and how would you describe body awareness to a friend?

_____
_____
_____

During your sessions, what are you most aware of?

_____
_____
_____

What are the advantages of developing your body awareness?

_____
_____

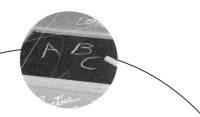

Client education tip 1.1

Help increase your client's body awareness by asking them a few simple awareness questions. For instance, ask him/her what side of the bed he/she sleeps on, which leg he/she lifts first when putting on a pair of pants or which arm he/she uses first when putting on a jacket. Awareness questions assist your client in becoming more self-observant and thus more self-reliant.

Self-observation 1.1

Getting to know you

Freeze your current reading position. You may be sitting, standing or lying down. Whatever your position is - hold it for a few moments.

Notice your overall position.
Are you standing, sitting, lying down or in some other position?
Is this your common reading position?

Notice the position of your back.
Does this position feel familiar to you?
Is your back comfortable?
Does it feel tense?

Notice the position of your legs and feet.
Does this position feel familiar to you?
Are your legs crossed?
Are your feet in contact with the ground?
Are your legs and feet comfortable?
Are your feet falling asleep?

Notice the position of your shoulders and arms.
Is this a common position for them?
Are you shoulders comfortable?
Are you holding your shoulders up, down, forward or backward?

Notice how you are holding this book.
Are you using your hands to hold it or are you using something else?
Are you holding it with both hands or just one?
If your hands aren't holding the book, what are they doing?
Are your hands comfortable or stiff?

Notice the position of your head.
Are you holding it up or down?
Are you holding it to the right or left?
Is this how you normally hold your head when reading?

continued

Notice the sensations in your neck.
Does your neck feel comfortable?
Does it feel tense and contracted?

Finally, notice how you are breathing.
Are you breathing deeply or shallowly?
Are you breathing primarily from your chest?
Are you breathing from your abdomen?
Does your current reading position allow you to breathe freely?

Now stop holding your reading position and move around, taking a few deep breaths.

Develop an awareness of yourself in everyday situations, e.g., notice how you sit when reading a book or how you stand when talking to a friend. In general, this will help develop body awareness, and will lead the way to develop a more specific awareness of your body mechanics as a manual therapist.

Self-feedback
What did you notice regarding your back, legs and feet, shoulders and arms, head and neck and breathing?

_____

_____

_____

Did you notice anything about your reading posture that surprised you?

_____

_____

_____

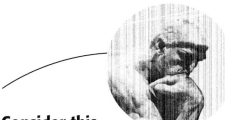

Consider this

"Awareness is the part of the consciousness which involves knowledge." [2]

Dr. Moshe Feldenkrais

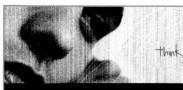

Something to think about...

Describe a few of your "good habits".

_____

_____

_____

_____

_____

Describe a few of your "bad habits".

_____

_____

_____

_____

_____

What habits come to mind when you think about your body mechanics?

_____

_____

_____

_____

_____

Describe a movement habit from your everyday life that you have transferred into your body mechanics.

_____

_____

_____

_____

_____

_____

_____

_____

Movement habits

We learn and form habits from the beginning of life and continue the process until we die. Some even say that the process of learning habits begins before birth. Knight Dunlap, in his book "Habits: Their Making and Unmaking", writes "the process of learning is the formation of a habit", and "a habit is a way of living that has been learned."[3] As we learn and accumulate our habits, it becomes clear that some habits serve us well, while others do not. "Bad habits" are considered harmful, while "good habits" are praised.

As you develop your body awareness, you can begin to become aware of your habits of movement. Movement habits are patterns of movement you repeat over and over again - often without being aware that you are actually using them. For example, the way you move when you walk, the posture you hold when standing and how you gesture when you talk are all elements of your movement habits. As creatures of habit, we transfer movement patterns and habits from one moment to the next and from one environment to another.

In _Self-observation 1.1_, you had the opportunity to become aware of your reading position. You may have discovered certain positions that seemed familiar to you, like the position of your back, legs, shoulders or head. As mentioned before, most of your movements and postures are habitual and you reuse them over and over again.

Action Once more, freeze your position and notice how similar your position is now, compared to the last time you froze. Even though you have walked or moved around since _Self-observation 1.1_, it's highly probable that you are still in a relatively similar position!

As a manual therapist, you transfer many of your everyday movement habits into your working environment. These are habits of movement you integrate into your practice of manual therapy and that, for whatever reason, you repeat over and over. For example, the way you sit when interviewing a new client may be the same way that you sit when eating dinner or the way you breathe when applying pressure may be the same way that you breathe when pushing a heavy object. Becoming aware of your habitual movement patterns and understanding how you integrate them into your body mechanics continues your development of awareness. In the next section you will learn how to sense which of your movement habits serve you and which ones hinder and cause you discomfort, pain or injury.

Self-observation 1.2

Transferring movement habits

Stand as if you were going to talk to a friend whom you just happened to meet at the store.

While standing, answer the following questions:
Note: *If, for some reason, you cannot answer some of the questions, don't worry – these are only a few of many possible observations. There may be things you notice that are not asked here. If so, write them below in the space provided.*

Are you balanced on both feet equally?
Are you standing on one foot?
Which foot do you primarily stand on, your right or your left?
Do you tend to stand still or do you shift your weight from one foot to the other?

Are you bearing more weight on one hip?
Are you standing with one hip rotated backward or forward?

Are both knees straight or slightly bent?
Is one knee straight and the other bent?

Is your back in a neutral position?
Is your back bent forward or backward?

Are your shoulders relaxed or are they held up, down, forward or backward?
Do you cross your arms in front of your chest or abdomen?
Are your hands in your pockets?
Are you holding a hand on your hip?

Is your head tilted to one side?
Are you looking to the right or left of your friend's face or at the middle?

What is the quality of your breathing?
Are you holding your breath?
Are you breathing deeply or shallowly?

Rest.

continued

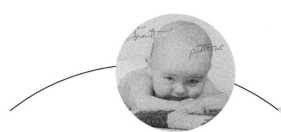

Consider this

As a baby, you developed movement patterns and habits that eventually evolved into the patterns and habits you have today. Research has shown that beginning from the age of two months, a baby is forming patterns that include the movements of the eyes. From the age of two months on, the baby forms movement patterns including facial expressions, sleeping position, vocal patterns and hand gestures. By the age of 2-3 years, the child is a "creature of habit".[4]

Walk around and shake yourself out.
Now stand beside your therapy table, as if you were going to work with a client.

While standing, answer these familiar questions:
Are you balanced on both feet equally?
Are you standing on one foot?
Which foot do you primarily stand on, your right or your left?
Do you tend to stand still or do you shift your weight from one foot to the other?

Are you bearing more weight on one hip?
Are you standing with one hip rotated back or forward?

Are both knees straight or slightly bent?
Is one knee straight and the other bent?

Is your back in a neutral position?
Is your back bent forward or backward?

Are your shoulders relaxed or are they held up, down, backward or forward?
Do you cross your arms in front of your chest or abdomen?
Are your hands in your pockets?
Are you holding a hand on your hip?

Do you rotate or tilt your head to one side?

What is the quality of your breathing?
Are you holding your breath?
Are you breathing deeply or shallowly?

Become more aware of your everyday life movement habits to help recognize which ones you transfer to your body mechanics as a manual therapist.

Self-feedback
What standing habits transferred from one situation to the next?

_____

_____

Were you aware of these habits or did you discover something new?

_____

Which habits did you find comfortable and which would you choose to change?

_____

_____

_____

Ease vs. effort–your skeleton

Once you become more aware of your body and movement habits, you can begin to discover which movement habits serve you and which ones hinder and cause you discomfort, pain or injury. Therefore, it is important to learn why some habits of movement feel easy and why some require effort.

How we use our musculoskeletal system in gravity is a significant factor as to why some movements feel easy and some more difficult. The reality is, gravity is a powerful force which our body must contend with. Realizing that gravity can be used to our advantage is a crucial part of developing effective and effortless body mechanics. When you work with gravity, instead of against it, flexibility, endurance, balance and sensitivity are increased.[5]

Using gravity to our advantage sounds fine, but how does one manage it? The good news is, our skeleton is designed to support our body to endure the force of gravity - it does this best when used optimally, for example, when vertically aligned.[6] When the skeleton is vertically aligned, all of the bones are "stacked", one on top of the other, in such a way that they can endure up to 2000 pounds of atmospheric pressure.[7] In this case, the skeleton is being used as it was intended, for support. The postural muscles can then be used more effectively to move your body with ease and comfort.

However, when the skeleton is not used optimally, for example, when standing with the spine bent forward, the back muscles must compensate to accommodate the skeleton's lack of support.[8] This scenario causes a sense of effort in your body mechanics and ultimately causes discomfort and pain in your body.

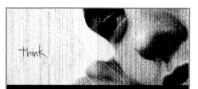

think

Something to think about...

Think of a situation where your body mechanics felt effortless?

_____

_____

In the above situation, were you using gravity to your advantage? If so, explain.

_____

_____

_____

_____

_____

_____

Now think of a situation where your body mechanics felt difficult and strained.

_____

_____

_____

_____

_____

_____

In the above situation were you using gravity to your disadvantage? If so, explain.

_____

_____

_____

_____

_____

_____

_____

_____

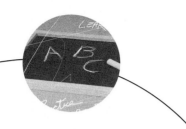

Client education tip 1.2

Show your clients a picture of the skeleton and give them a visual and kinesthetic sense of the shape and strength of their skeleton. If appropriate, lead them through Partner practice 1.1. Many clients are in "skeletal denial" and don't fully under-stand what their skeleton looks like and why they have one.

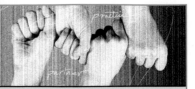

Partner practice 1.1

The strength of bone

Sit on a chair with your feet slightly in back of or in front of your knees. Ask your partner to slowly sit down on one of your knees. (See figure 1.1)

Notice how your leg responds to your partner's weight.
Does your partner feel heavy?
Can you feel your leg muscles working hard to support her/his weight?
What sensations do you feel in your knee and ankle joints?

Notice if there is a change in your breathing while you support your partner in this manner.
Are you breathing quickly or shallowly?

Now ask your partner to stand up. Move your leg so that your ankle and heel are now under your knee. Ask your partner to sit on your knee again. (See figure 1.2)

Notice how your leg responds to your partner's weight now.
Does she/he feel lighter than before?
Are your leg muscles working less to support his/her weight?
Can you sense that the bones of your leg are easily supporting your partner's weight?
Are your knee and ankle joints more comfortable?

Is there a change in your breathing now that your bones are supporting your partner's weight?
Are you breathing more normally?

When working, keep the kinesthetic experience of this lesson in mind. This memory will help reinforce the importance of utilizing the strength of your bones.

Partner feedback
How secure did your partner feel when sitting on your leg the first time? _____
How secure did your partner feel the second time?

_____
How can you use the strength of your bones to improve your body mechanics?

_____

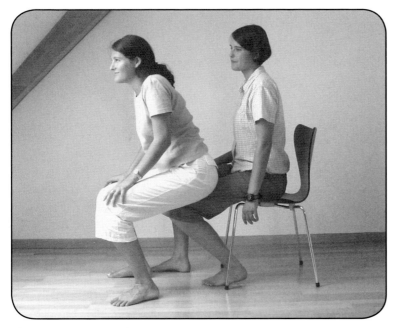

Figure 1.1

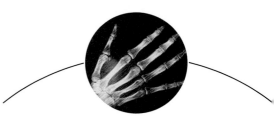

Practice tip 1.2

During your sessions try the following:

Visualize your skeleton, from head to toe.

Become aware of the strength of your bones.

Sense where your skeleton is vertically aligned and where it is not.

Let your skeleton support you.

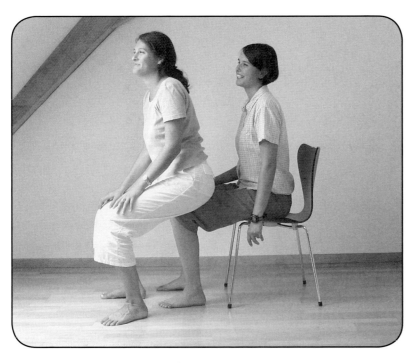

Figure 1.2

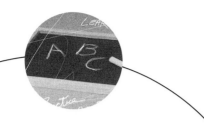

Ease vs. effort–your muscles

Your skeletal or postural muscles, for example, your pectoralis major, latisimus dorsi, biceps brachii, gluteus medius, quadriceps, hamstrings and gastrocnemius are voluntary muscles that keep you moving despite the force of gravity. The fact that they are voluntary means you have control over their quality of movement.

When your postural muscles are used in a balanced and well-organized manner, you have a sense of ease and comfort in your movements. The larger muscles, for example, the muscles of the pelvis and legs, are allowed to work in a powerful way and the smaller muscles, for example, the muscles of the shoulder girdle and arm, are allowed to perform skillful and refined work.[10]

An imbalanced use of your postural muscles can lead to areas of tightness and contraction, and often cause your skeleton to become misaligned due to the accompanying imbalance.[11] For example, frequently lifting with the smaller muscles of your upper body instead of using the larger, stronger muscles of your lower body manifests a sense of effort and discomfort in your body mechanics. Eventually, this can lead to fatigue of the smaller muscles, abnormal holding patterns, pain or injury.

When you are using your musculoskeletal system optimally, your skeleton can support you and your postural muscles can remain free to move without excessive effort. Furthermore, becoming aware of which movement habits in your body mechanics require effort and which ones feel easy and comfortable will greatly increase your overall body awareness and will consequently prevent injury.

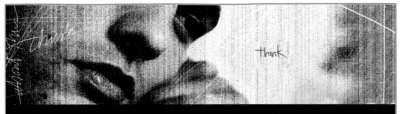

Something to think about...

Think of a situation where you felt your postural muscles were working in a balanced and well-organized manner.

_____
_____
_____
_____
_____

In the above situation, how did the performance of your postural muscles affect the quality of your body mechanics?

_____
_____
_____
_____
_____

Now think of a situation where you felt your postural muscles were working in an imbalanced manner.

_____
_____
_____
_____
_____

How did the above situation affect the quality of your body mechanics?

_____
_____
_____
_____
_____

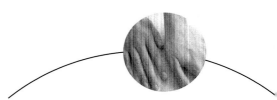

Practice tip 1.3

During your sessions try the following:

When you feel comfortable with your body mechanics, notice if you are using less effort. When you begin to feel uncomfortable with your body mechanics, notice if you are using too much effort.

Ease vs. effort

Put an object that weighs about 10 to15 pounds on a table. Stand next to the object and pick it up.
(See figure 1.3)

Notice if the object feels easy or difficult to pick up.
Does it feel light or heavy?

Notice how your body responds to picking up the object.
Do you feel comfortable picking it up from this distance?
Are you straining any muscles?
Is your skeleton aligned?
Can you breathe comfortably?

Put the object down and rest for a moment.
Now stand a few inches away from the object and pick it up again. **(See figure 1.4)**

From this distance, is the object easier or more difficult to pick up?
Does it feel heavy or light?

Notice how your body responds to picking up the object.
Do you feel comfortable picking it up from this distance?
Are you straining any muscles?
Is your skeleton misaligned?
Can you breathe comfortably?

Put the object down and rest for a moment.
Once more, stand next to the object and pick it up.

Again, notice how your body responds when picking up the object from this closer distance.

Discovering what it feels like to use your musculoskeletal system in a well-balanced manner will help you develop an awareness of body mechanics that allows you to feel the difference between ease vs. effort.

Self-feedback
In which standing position was it easier to pick up the object? _____
Why was it easier in this position? _____
_____

How can you better use your musculoskeletal system to create a sense of ease and use less effort in your body mechanics?
_____
_____

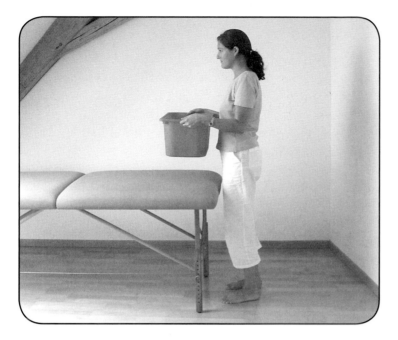

Figure 1.3

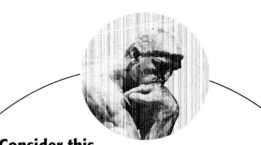

Consider this

"Good posture is an easy, balanced position of the body that does not place excessive stresses upon the tissues of the body." [12]

Dr. Joseph E. Muscolino

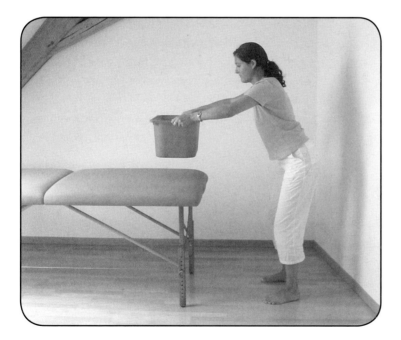

Figure 1.4

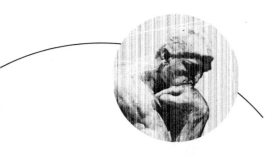

Consider this

Do you remember Randy Newman's song "Short People" and the ever-so popular line "Short people got no reason to live."? Well listen up, Mr. Newman...

As it turns out, a short person is less likely to fall than a tall person is. Here's why:

The center of gravity of an object, including a person, is the point where the weight of the object is concentrated. An object is stable when its center of gravity is located over its base. The lower an object's center of gravity is compared to its height, the less likely it is to fall over. This ability to resist falling over is called "mechanical stability" and the height of a person affects their mechanical stability. Generally speaking, a shorter person has a lower center of gravity, giving them greater mechanical stability than that of a tall person.[9]

Awareness of choice

In *Self-observation 1.3*, you had the opportunity to sense the difference between ease and effort. If you had the chance to pick up the object again, which position would you choose – standing a few inches away or standing close? If you chose the closer, easier and more comfortable distance, congratulations! You now have a sense of effortless and easy body mechanics.

Developing body awareness, by identifying your movement and postural habits and sensing the difference between ease and effort, leads to an awareness of choice. Having a choice, no matter the situation, gives you a sense of freedom and ultimately improves your quality of life.

Moshe Feldenkrais, founder of the Feldenkrais Method®, believed that your advantage as a human being is your ability to perform the same act in at least three different ways; three options are the minimum and will guarantee greater efficiency, giving you the feeling that you are a free person and the master of your life.[13] In relation to your body mechanics, this awareness of options allows you to develop a wide range of easy, comfortable, effective and dynamic alternatives for any given movement. For example, becoming aware of how comfortable you are when lifting your client's head and, if you find that you are not comfortable, exploring easier and more effective alternatives. Over time, if you develop your awareness of choice and exercise it on a regular basis, you will use problematic movement habits less and develop a vast repertoire of efficient options, creating a sense of freedom and ease in your body mechanics.

As mentioned in the beginning of this chapter, there is no quick fix that will automatically give you pain-free and perfect body mechanics. Developing sound body mechanics is an ongoing process. By studying this book, you will soon be on your way to gaining an inner wisdom that will yield a solid self-care strategy, effective and dynamic body mechanics and longevity of practice.

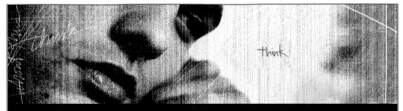

Something to think about...

When you think of "awareness of choice", what comes to mind and how would you describe it to a friend.

_____
_____
_____

Describe your repertoire of body mechanics and how you have developed it.

_____
_____
_____
_____
_____
_____

What are the advantages of developing a wide range of body mechanics alternatives? _____

_____
_____
_____
_____

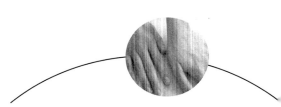

Practice tip 1.4

During your sessions try the following:

Pick a movement habit, for example, how you use your hands to apply pressure, and see if you can find at least 2 alternatives. This will help you become more aware of your choices and begin the process of developing a wide range of possible movements, making your sessions more creative and interesting for you and your clients.

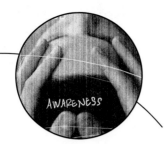

Consider This

"To foster inner awareness, introspection and reasoning is more efficient than meditation and prayer." [14]

HH Dalai Lama

Summary

Body awareness

Self-care begins with developing body awareness. Body awareness is a mindfulness of your body's movements, responses, sensations and feelings. As you develop this mindfulness, you become more aware of subtle movement patterns. Developing body awareness requires you to become more self-observant, not only when you are performing manual therapy, but also during your everyday life.

Movement habits

Once you become aware of your body, you can begin to become aware of your movement habits. Movement habits are patterns we re-peat over and over again. We need habits in order to live and because all of us are creatures of habit, we cannot help but transfer movement patterns and habits from one moment to the next and from one en-vironment to another. As a manual therapist, you transfer many of your lifelong and everyday movement patterns and habits into your working environment through your body mechanics.

Ease vs. effort

When you are using your musculoskeletal system optimally, your skeleton can support you and your postural muscles can remain free to move without excessive effort. Furthermore, becoming aware of which movement habits in your body mechanics require effort and which ones feel easy and comfortable will greatly increase your over-all body awareness and will consequently prevent injury.

Awareness of choice

Developing body awareness, by identifying your movement habits and sensing the difference between ease and effort, leads to an awareness of choice. Over time, if you develop your awareness of choice and ex-ercise it on a regular basis, you will use problematic movement habits less and develop a vast repertoire of efficient options, creating a sense of freedom and ease in your body mechanics.

Now that you've read this chapter...

How would you rate your body awareness?

always aware   mostly aware   sometimes aware   not very aware

What part of your body are you most aware of?
- upper body
- lower body
- head
- other_____

What aspects of your body mechanics do you feel most comfortable with?
- standing
- sitting
- applying pressure
- other_____

Describe 5 movement habits that you are aware of using during every session.

1. _____
2. _____
3. _____
4. _____
5. _____

Describe a specific part of your body mechanics that feels easy and comfortable.

_____
_____

Describe a specific part of your body mechanics that feels difficult and uncomfortable.

_____
_____

How satisfied are you with your understanding of body awareness in relation to your body mechanics?
- 100%
- 75%
- 50%
- 25%

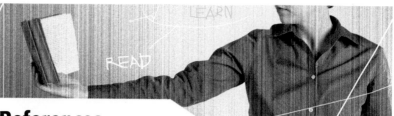

References

1.   Watson D. A *Report into the Demographic Incidence of Wrist and Finger Damage to Bodywork Practitioners.* Shi'Zen Publications. 2000.

2.   Rosenfield, Edward. *The Forebrain: Sleep, Consciousness, Awareness and Learning: An Interview with Moshe Feldenkrais.* Interface Journal, Nos. 3-4, 1976.

3.   Dunlap, Knight. *Habits: The Making and Unmaking.* New York: Liveright, 1972.

4.   Begley, Sharon. *The Nature of Nurturing.* Newsweek Special Magazine. March 2000.

5.   Park, Glen. *A New Approach to The Alexander Technique: Moving Toward a More Balanced Expression of the Whole Self.* California: The Crossing Press, 1998.

6.   Rolf, Ida P. *Rolfing: Reestablishing the Natural Alignment and Structural Integration of the Human Body.* Rochester: Healing Arts Press, 1989.

7.   Chester, John. *Personal Communication.* Feldenkrais Professional Training Program. Seattle, WA, 1999.

8.   Todd, Mabel E. *The Thinking Body.* Brooklyn: Dance Horizons/Princeton Book Co., 1979.

9.   VanCleave, Janice. *Center of Gravity: Tilted; Science for Fun; Science Fair Central;* DiscoverySchool.com. www.school.discovery.com. 15 March 2003.

10. Haller, Jeff. Feldenkrais Professional Training Program. Maui, Hawaii, 1994.

11. Rolf, Ida P. R*olfing: Integration of Human Structures.* New York: Harper Row, 1977.

12. Muscolino, Joseph E. *Electronic Communication.* June 2003.

13. Alon, Ruthy. *Mindful Spontaneity: Moving in Tune with Nature.* England: Prism Press, 1990.

14. Singh, Renuka. *The Dalai Lama's Book of Daily Meditations.* London: Rider, 1999.

2 *Outside Basics*

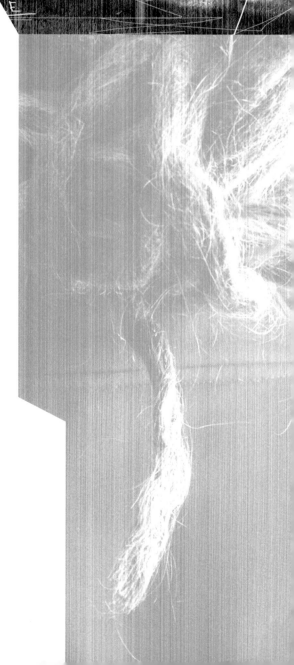

Introduction

Before we discuss the more common topics of body mechanics, such as how to lift and bend properly, let's look at some of the not so common topics. The next two chapters include such topics as lighting, space, breathing and hydration. These, and many others, are the "basic" elements of your body mechanics, and are important to consider when building a successful self-care strategy.

This chapter includes specific topics concerning your "outside" basics. The outside basics are elements of your external working environment and important to keep in mind before and during your sessions.

Discussed are different aspects of therapy tables and chairs, and guidelines to consider when purchasing them. Lighting, space, floor coverings, clothes, shoes, hair and nails are also discussed, giving you key points to become more aware of.

Before you read this chapter...

How would you rate your awareness of your working environment?

always aware   mostly aware   sometimes aware   not very aware

What part of your surroundings are you most aware of?

- spatial
- visual
- tactile (what you physically touch)
- other_____

What part of your surroundings are you least aware of ?

- spatial
- visual
- tactile
- other_____

Describe 5 aspects of your surroundings. (e.g., furniture, lighting, decoration)

1. _____
2. _____
3. _____
4. _____
5. _____

Describe an aspect of your surroundings that you enjoy and feel comfortable with.

_____
_____

Describe an aspect of your surroundings that you dislike and would like to change.

_____
_____

How satisfied are you with your surroundings?

- completely
- mostly
- a little
- not at all

Tables

Developing a self-care strategy not only involves taking care of your body, but also includes choosing a table of the utmost quality. Like your body, your table is one of your most important tools. Therefore, careful thought and scrupulous attention should be given when choosing your table.

First, ask yourself whether you need a portable or a stationary table. The fact is, many manual therapists buy a portable table but never actually carry it. Be honest with yourself - will you move your table from place to place or will you work in one location. If you are going to move your table around, then buy a portable table. However, if you plan on working in one location, then consider buying a stationary table.

In regards to your body mechanics, an electric table is the best choice. An electric table gives you the ability to adjust your table height effortlessly, allowing you to work with your client at the required height. Body mechanics are often compromised when therapists find that their table height is not optimal, and yet, for many reasons, continue working without making adjustments. Recently, many advances have been made in the development of electric tables and today there are several models to choose from, at a relatively low cost. The bottom line is: an electric table saves you the inconvenience of having to manually adjust your table (or disturb your client to do so in the middle of a session), and most importantly, supports healthy body mechanics - you have the choice to raise or lower your table at any time, ensuring the best use of body weight and leverage.

Finally, when considering a table, spend time examining the details. Look at the quality of each individual component, for example, wood, braces, cables, screws, padding, leg extensions and face rests, and then examine how they are all put together to support each other in performance.

Consumer tip 2.1

Be sure to ask what kinds of manufacture performance tests have been made on the table, for example, tests for dynamic load, lateral force and stability. Make sure the table has a lifetime warranty and read the fine print - many companies convert their "lifetime warranty" to a 5-year warranty upon discontinuing a model.

Here are specific points to keep in mind:

Strength: Your table should be able to support, not only the weight of your client, but your weight as well. If you choose to get on your table to work, you need to feel absolutely secure in knowing that your table can support your additional weight and movements.

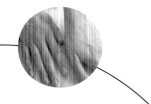

Practice tip 2.1

Many injuries have occurred while transporting tables. Don't be in a rush to get your table, for example, up the stairs or into your car. Take your time and be mindful of your body mechanics.

Consumer tip 2.2

Ask a friend, sales representative or willing bystander to lie down on each table you are considering and then get on the table with them. Spend a few minutes working with them as if they were a client. Make sure both of you feel totally comfortable with the table's ability to hold your combined weight and movements.

Stability: Like strength, the stability of your table is also a crucial point. The table you choose should give you full peace of mind knowing it will withstand the specific nuances of your work. For example, if you compress, push and pull, jostle, rock or bounce, there should be no doubt in your mind that your table will remain stable. Your table should also remain sturdy during the movements of your client. For instance, if your client sits on the end of or leans up against your table, you want to be absolutely sure that it will not, in the slightest way, buckle.

Consumer tip 2.3

Often body mechanics are compromised because of a table's instability. For example, if a table's top is too flexible, the practitioner must make up for this lack of resistance by pressing harder with her hands. Consider purchasing a table with a w/4mm plywood top or "reinforcing ribs" or ideally, both. These elements increase a table's stability and reduce table top flexibility, allowing your body, especially your hands, the freedom to do the delicate and refined work of manual therapy, without working hard.

Comfort: A strong and stable table will certainly add to your peace of mind and to your client's comfort, but it is the material on which they rest that leaves a lasting impression. Make sure your table is sufficiently padded and the covering material is soft and easy to clean. Your tabletop should give your client a nurturing cushion of support that, added to the strength and stability of your table, allows them to fully relax and enjoy your work.

Consumer tip 2.4

Are you surprised to learn that there are many therapists who have never actually lain down on their own table? Spend as much time as needed to experience the qualities of comfort boasted by the table manufacturer of your consideration. Lie prone, using the face cradle-could you rest comfortably there for an hour? Notice if there is adequate space to rest your arms in both prone and supine positions. Make sure the padding provides not only a solid foundation, but also a generous cushion of comfort, in general, higher-density foams support better and wear longer. Ultimately, you need to ask yourself if you would feel comfortable receiving a session on the table you are considering.

A few last, but equally important points:

Make sure the face cradle is fashioned in such a way that you can get as close to your client as possible.

The height of your table should be easily adjustable to your specific needs. Make sure that the leg extensions attach to the legs in a strong and sturdy way.

If you are considering an electric table, the motor should be powerful and relatively quiet.

Your table should be wide enough to accommodate many body types comfortably, yet narrow enough to ensure effective body mechanics.

If you transport your table, use a carrying case and/or cart that support your body mechanics. Make sure the carrying straps are positioned in such a way that they fit you effectively and comfortably.

If you have special requirements, buy a table that can accommodate most, if not all of them. A prenatal table should be considered if you practice pregnancy massage. If you work with athletes, consider a table with extensions for length and additional built-in support for sports massage and deeper work. Consider a table with extra features such as a tilting back and elevating legs if you specialize in injury and rehabilitation work. If a large percentage of your clients are women, consider a table with breast recesses.

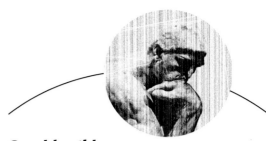

Consider this

"While some of your treatments will be on larger clients, all of your treatments have to accommodate you. If a table is too wide, you reduce that angle at which you apply your body weight through your shoulders to your arms and hands. This loss of efficiency may not be felt if you're doing just one or two treatments per day. But if you have a busy practice, you are likely to experience more fatigue than you would if you could step in closer." [1]

Tim Herbert, CustomCraftworks

Table Height

Your table should be set at a height that allows you to use your body weight rather than excessive muscular effort. If your table is too high for the required treatment, then your shoulders and upper body will be strained, and if your table is too low, then your lower back will suffer.

The kind of treatments you execute will determine your table height. In general, your table should be set lower for deep work, mid-thigh for relaxation work and higher for light work. These heights take into consideration your height, the depth of the client's body and allow you to use your body weight. If you find that you need to adjust your table once you begin your treatment and you do not have an electric table, don't hesitate to stop and adjust it. Many therapists do not take the time to make height adjustments between or during sessions. However, to support healthy body mechanics, it is worth taking the time to make the adjustment. If you are in the middle of a session, if needed, wrap your client up in a sheet or towel and help them up.

Note: Not having to disturb your client to make a height adjustment is an excellent reason for considering an electric table.

With that said, there is no "correct" height for everyone. It is important for you to discover what is the best table height for your body type, i.e., one person can have a long torso and short legs, while another has a short torso and long legs. If an instructor or colleague prefers or recommends a "lower" table, make sure a "lower" table is right for you. Don't assume that someone else knows what is the best table height for your body type and techniques.

If you primarily sit to work, your table should be at a height where your upper body does not need to strain in order to work with your client. Working with your table above your knees allows you to sit close and bend, push and pull from your hip joints. If your table height is such that it meets your knees, you may have the tendency to sit with your legs spread too far apart in order to get close enough to your client. This posture can strain the low back and compromise your effectiveness.

Consumer tip 2.5

If you mainly sit to work, consider an "access panel". These arched panels at the head and foot end of the tables allow you to sit closer to your client.

Chairs and stools

Like your body and table, your chair or stool is also an important tool and should be chosen carefully. At first glance, it may not seem like such a big concern, but if your chair or stool does not fully support you, over time you will start to feel the negative effects in your body, compromising your energy level and effectiveness.

It is up to you whether you choose a chair or a stool. Over the last few years, stools have become more popular, but you should choose what surface feels the most comfortable and right for you. In general, a chair or stool that gives you firm support is the best choice. A chair or stool with firm support allows your pelvis and thighs to maintain clear contact with its surface. A chair with a soft and cushy surface does not give the firm resistance that your pelvis and thighs need to maintain their contact with the surface. At first, a soft, cushioned surface feels great, but in a few minutes your skeletal support gives way to your muscular body and soon your vertical alignment is sinking downward. This doesn't mean to imply that you must sit on a slab of cement. Simply choose a chair or stool which will solidly support you in all aspects of your work.

Stability: Your chair or stool should be strong and stable. If you should decide to stand on your chair or stool during your treatment, you want to be certain that it will hold your weight and support your movements.

Consumer tip 2.6

Don't hesitate to test the stability of the chair or stool in question. Sit on it and move around a bit. Make sure that it does not wobble. Listen for any sound that might indicate that the chair or stool has weaknesses. Also, don't be embarrassed to further test its stability by standing on it.

Mobility: You should be able to easily move your chair or stool from one place to the next. If your chair is heavy, picking it up to move it may impede your body mechanics. Chairs and stools that are equipped with rollers are easier to move around, just make sure that your floor covering does not hamper your movements.

If the chair or stool you are considering does not have rollers, pick it up and carry it around – as you would during a session with a client. Get a sense of how heavy it is and if its weight is such that you can manage it throughout your working day. (It may feel relatively light at first, but can you realistically pick it up and put it down all day long?) If the chair or stool of your choice has rollers, spend some time rolling around on it. Can you easily maneuver it around? Test the chair's ability to roll over floor coverings similar to what your have in your office. And finally, is it relatively quiet when rolling or does it sound like a truck rolling across the floor?

Comfort: Make sure the surface size of the chair or stool accommodates your body type. If the surface is too small, you will not feel stable. The surface edge should be well-rounded so that it does not press sharply into the back of your legs. This can cause an impingement of the sciatic nerve, resulting in pain and numbness. Chairs and stools that are equipped with an adjustable height feature are convenient and help you maintain a comfortable height at all times.

Sit on the chair or stool and feel if it suits your body type. This is easier said than done. The construction of most chairs and stools do not take into consideration the difference in body types. However, this does not mean you need to settle for less than a comfortable surface. If you are unable to find a chair or stool that accommodates your body, then consider a bench-type surface. This option will give you more surface room. Make sure the surface edge of the chair or stool does not press into the back of your legs.

A few more important points:

Chairs with back support are fine. Just make sure the back support is secure and does not automatically tilt back when you lean against it. As with the surface of your chair, you want the back support to give you firm support.

The height of the chair or stool should allow your knees to be at the same height as your hips and allow your feet to rest flat on the floor.

Have a chair or stool available for yourself even if you do not sit to work. You never know when you might need to use it. This also gives your client the choice to sit before, during and after his/her treatment.

Space

Environmental space engineers believe that your space can affect your mood and behavior.[2]

In a situation where space is restricted, not only are your mood and behavior potentially affected in a negative way, but so are your body mechanics. In this case, your body mechanics can become restricted, giving you the sense that you must conserve your range of movements and adapt yourself to the limited space. You need enough room to move around your table or other working surfaces freely. If you are concerned, consciously or unconsciously, about bumping into a wall or nearby object, you cannot give your total attention to your work.

On the other hand, when you have adequate work space around you, your body mechanics are less likely to be restricted, giving you the sense that you can move freely around your table or other working surfaces without hesitating.

However, not all work situations are ideal or flexible. If your situation is such that you don't have quite enough space, the best thing to do is adapt to the space available. If possible, clear the room of all unnecessary furniture and items taking up space and place your table so it has equal space around all sides. Becoming aware of your space limitation and how it affects your quality of therapy can make all the difference. Increasing your awareness can change your mood, attention, breath and movements within your space, regardless of the quantity of space available.

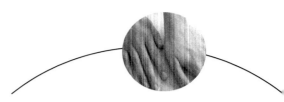

Practice tip 2.2

How much space do you have in your therapy room? The next time you enter your room, take a few minutes and look around. Get a sense of the space around your table, as well as the arrangement of the furniture and adornments. Are you using your space effectively? Are there some changes that you would like to make? If so, take the time and make them.

Something to think about...

Think about the last time you were in a situation where you felt as though you didn't have enough space around you, for example, eating in a restaurant, standing in an elevator or sitting in a plane.

How did the lack of space affect your mood, behavior, breathing and movements?

_____

_____

_____

Now think about the last time you were in a situation where you felt as though you had all the space required to feel comfortable and at ease. How did having enough space affect your mood, behavior, breathing and movements?

_____

_____

_____

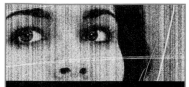
Lighting

In general, lighting should be bright enough for you to see what you are doing clearly. If the lighting is too low, your eyes will need to strain to see. When your eyes are strained, a chain reaction starts from your head down to your feet: your head and neck fall forward, your spine and pelvis follow, and your legs and feet lose their stability. Over time, this kind of reaction can cause discomfort in your body mechanics. When your lighting level is such that you can clearly see what you are doing, your body mechanics are less likely to suffer due to eye strain.

In some cases, for example working in a softly lit spa, having the option to change the lighting level may not seem possible. However, if you feel your current lighting level is not adequate for your needs but is used by management to create a therapeutic atmosphere, there may be creative alternatives possible. You could, for example, suggest clients wear eye covers similar to those handed out by airlines to block out light. Remember, when your comfort level is compromised, so is the comfort of your client.

Floor coverings

Area rugs are wonderful for adding warmth and texture, but they can be problematic. If an area rug is underneath or near your table, make sure it does not get in the way of your movement. It is easy to trip or become distracted by a rug. Keep it secured to the floor so it does not bunch up or cause you to interrupt your movement. Also, an area rug could be hazardous to a client who is trying to maneuver around an unfamiliar room. Rolling a chair over a rug can be difficult, thus distracting you from your session. Again, secure the rug so it stays in place while you and your client are moving around your space.

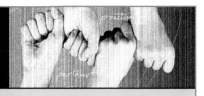

Partner practice 2.1

Lighting your way

Ask your partner to lie down on your table, as if you were beginning a session together.
Adjust your lighting level such that it gives you adequate light to see what you are doing clearly.
Begin to work with your partner and become aware of how your body mechanics respond to having enough light in which to work.

Sense the comfort level in your eyes.

Do you feel your eyes straining to see? (If not, then this is a good lighting level. If yes, then try adjusting the light so that your eyes do not need to strain.)

Now adjust the lighting level so that you can sense the difference between an adequate level and a level that is too low. For a few moments, work with your partner using a lighting level that is obviously too low, and become aware of how your body mechanics respond to not having enough light in which to work.

Sense the strain on your eyes.

How does the rest of your body respond to the current strain on your eyes?
How does your neck compensate for your eye strain?
How do your back, pelvis, legs and feet compensate for your eye stain?

Now adjust the lighting back to an adequate level. Again, work with your partner.

Notice how quickly your body mechanics respond to a comfortable lighting level.

Though it is a very subtle element of your body mechanics, proper lighting increases your comfort level, as well as your client's.

Partner feedback

How did your body mechanics respond to the different levels of lighting?

_____

How did your partner experience your touch when using inadequate light?

_____

How did your partner experience your touch when using adequate light?

_____

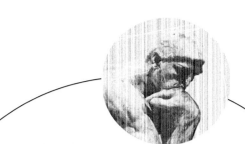

Consider this

The Greeks used pebble mosaics as floor coverings as early as the 8th century BC. Tessellated pavement (mosaics of regularly shaped cubes) show up in the Hellenistic Age and by the1st century AD had come into popular use in and around thermal baths throughout the Roman Empire. Inlaid stone, popular in Byzantine, Renaissance and Gothic architecture, is now popular in health spas all over the world.[3]

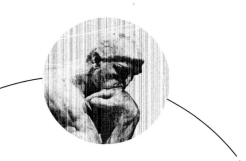

Clothing

Ideally, your clothing should not restrict or get in the way of your movement. Frequently stopping to rearrange your clothing is a sure sign of clothing interference, e.g., having to stop in the middle of a manipulation to roll up a sleeve or tuck in a shirt. If your clothes are too tight, your effectiveness and comfort will be reduced. Wearing clothes that allow you to move freely is optimal.

Two areas to pay particular attention to are the waist and the chest. Wearing anything tight around your waist can become irritating, negatively affecting your disposition, breathing and body mechanics. Pay attention to how pants or any waist-level fitting garment feels to you. Can you move freely without restriction and can you sit comfortably without sensing a tightening around your waist?

For women, wearing a bra that is restrictive can also negatively influence your disposition, breathing and body mechanics. Wearing an athletic bra designed for continuous movement is ideal, especially for women who are large-breasted.

Natural fibers, such as silk, wool, linen or cotton are the best to wear, allowing your skin to breathe as you work. Synthetic fibers, such as polyester or nylon do not allow your body to breathe fully and, in dry conditions, can cause electric sparks to fly between you and your client.

Something to think about...

Take a few minutes and think about the kind of clothing you wear during your work time. Do you wear clothing which is comfortable and allows you to move freely?

_____

Are you restricted in any way by your clothing?

_____

_____

Is there a certain type of clothing that you feel totally comfortable wearing?

_____

_____

_____

Shoes

If you choose to wear shoes, wearing comfortable and supportive shoes is important, especially if you stand frequently throughout your sessions. The comfort and support of your feet will reflect on your disposition, breathing and body mechanics. Therefore, in or out of shoes, your feet should feel relaxed and connected to the ground when working.

Wearing a pair of uncomfortable shoes not only affects your disposition and breathing, but also your body mechanics. A pair of troublesome shoes can negatively influence your body mechanics to the point of not being able to stand any longer. Ouch!

Wearing a pair of comfortable shoes allows your feet to relax and connect to the ground while working. Wearing non-slip shoes is also a good idea, especially on an uncarpeted floor. On the other hand, many therapists are comfortable working barefoot or in socks. This is fine as long as your feet remain relaxed. If, however, you find that your feet are constantly sore, wearing supportive shoes may be the answer. If you prefer to wear socks, make sure that you are on a non-slip floor.

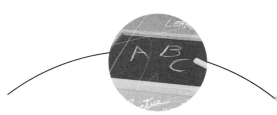

Client education tip 2.1

Tight waistbands and wallets carried in back pockets can exacerbate low back pain. Ask your clients if their waistbands are loose enough and suggest that wallets be carried elsewhere.

Client education tip 2.2

High-heeled shoes can potentially exacerbate back, leg and foot pain. Suggest low-heeled shoes to help alleviate discomfort. If your client has worn high-heeled shoes for a long time, suggest they adjust gradually to low-heeled shoes. (Some clients may be very attached to their particular shoe style, so be gently suggestive.)

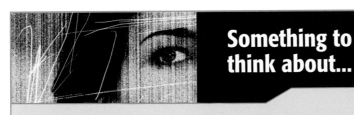

Something to think about...

Think about the last time you wore a pair of uncomfortable shoes, for example, a new pair of running, hiking or walking shoes. How did they affect your mood, behavior, breathing and movements?

_____

Now think about the last time you wore comfortable shoes. How did they affect your mood, behavior, breathing and movements?

_____

How do the shoes you are presently wearing feel?

_____

When working, what kind of shoes do you wear? Athletic? Walking? Sandals?

_____

How comfortable are your working shoes?

_____

Are your feet sore or relaxed after a day's work?

_____

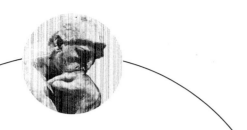

Consider this

If you have long hair and are thinking about cutting it, consider donating your hair to Locks of Love. Locks of Love is a non-profit organization providing hairpieces across the United States to financially disadvantaged children, 18 years and younger, suffering from long-term medical hair loss. You can contact them at www.locksoflove.org

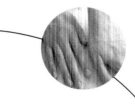

Practice tip 2.3

The next time your hair begins to distract you during a session, even if it is as simple as one strand falling into your face or getting into your eyes, notice how your body responds to the distraction. Once you remove the distraction, notice again how your body responds.

Hair

Hair control can make all the difference in the world when it comes to body mechanics. Whether short or long, if your hair is "out of control", so are your body mechanics.

Many therapists are not aware of how distracting their hair is until they find themselves holding their head, often unconsciously, to one side in order to keep their hair out of their face. This holding puts a tremendous strain on the muscles of the neck and back. If this habit persists, neck and/or back pain is likely to occur. Of course, all of this can be avoided with some awareness of hair control. The bottom line: keep your hair out of your face and prevent it from hanging down in front of you. Restrained hair is also hygienically prudent.

Nails

Believe it or not, the length of your nails can also affect your body mechanics. With short nails, there is no hesitancy to use the fingers or thumbs and the hand can work in a soft and relaxed fashion. With longer nails, the therapist is often concerned about scratching or hurting the client. This results in tense and less effective hand use. If your client can feel your nails, your nails are too long.

Being mindful of your nail length and keeping your nails short on a regular base will allow your hands to work in a flexible and supple manner. As with hair control, shorter nails are more hygienic.

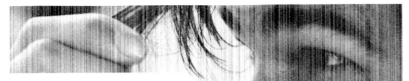

Summary

The outside basics are aspects of your external working environment and important to keep in mind before and during your sessions. Here is a review:

Like your body, your **table** is one of your most important tools. Therefore, careful forethought and scrupulous attention should be applied when choosing your table. Your **table** should be set at a **height** that allows you to use your body weight rather than excessive muscular effort. If your table is too high, your shoulders and upper body will be strained. If your table is too low, your low back will suffer. Like your body and table, your **chair or stool** is also an important tool and should be chosen carefully.

It is critical to have enough **space** to move around your table or other working surfaces freely, even if space is limited. In general, **lighting** should be bright enough for you to see what you are doing clearly. If the lighting is too low, your eyes will need to strain to see. **Area rugs** are wonderful for adding warmth and texture, but they can be problematic. If a rug or carpet is underneath or near your table, make sure it does not compromise your movements.

Ideally, your **clothing** should not distract you or restrict your movements. If you choose to wear **shoes**, wearing comfortable and supportive shoes is important, especially if you stand frequently throughout your sessions. **Hair** control can make all the difference in the world when it comes to body mechanics. Whether short or long, if your hair is out of control, so are your body mechanics. The length of your **nails** can also affect your body mechanics and the comfort of your client.

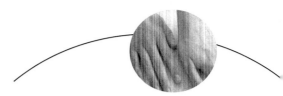

Practice tip 2.4

For client comfort, be especially mindful of your nail length when executing deep tissue work. Many therapists do not realize just how short their nails need to be, especially when working around bony areas, such as the scapula and suboccipital region.

Now that you've read this chapter...

How would you rate your awareness of your work surroundings?

⬤————————⬤————————⬤————————⬤

always aware　　*mostly aware*　　*sometimes aware*　　*not very aware*

What part of your surroundings were you most aware of?

○ *table height*
○ *space and lighting*
○ *clothes and shoes*
○ *other*_____

What part of your surroundings were you least aware of?

○ *table height*
○ *space and lighting*
○ *clothes and shoes*
○ *other*_____

Describe 5 aspects of your "outside basics".

1. _____
2. _____
3. _____
4. _____
5. _____

Describe an aspect of your "outside basics" that you enjoy and feel comfortable with.

_____
_____

Describe an aspect of your "outside basics" that you dislike and would like to change.

_____
_____

How satisfied are you with your understanding of the "outside basics"?

○ *100%*
○ *75%*
○ *50%*
○ *25%*

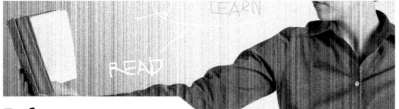

References

1. Herbert, Tim. *Electronic Communication.* May 2003.

2. Greiner, Lenore. *The Designs Are All-Inclusive; You Can Bank On It.* North County Times 9 May 2000. www.nctimes.net 24 July 2003.

3. Floor Covering. *Britannica Ready Reference.* Encyclopedia Britannica, Inc. 2001.

4. Flax. *Flax Council of Canada.* 15 September 2002. www.flaxcouncil.ca. 7 February 2003.

3 Inside Basics

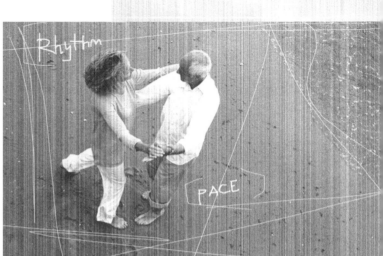

Introduction

When Shakespeare wrote the words, "To be or not to be", he was not referring to the physical demands on a manual therapist, but let us pretend, for a moment, he was. Manual therapy, no matter what type, is a very physically demanding profession. It requires you to have physical strength, endurance, flexibility, coordination and ingenuity. To maintain a practice that is healthy on all levels you must stay on "top of your game." Therefore, in order "to be", it is recommended that you incorporate the following "inside basics" into your self-care strategy.

Included in this chapter are topics such as warming up, resting, winding down, breathing, hydration, rhythm and pace. As you can see, these are the more internal or "inside" aspects of your working environment that, like the outside basics, are vital to keep in mind before, during and after your sessions. At the end of this chapter, you will have the opportunity to integrate the outside and inside basics into a *Partner practice* exercise. This will help you gain a better understanding of how to integrate the basics into your daily self-care strategy.

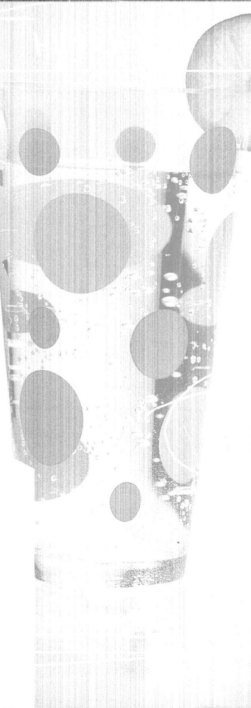

Before you read this chapter…

How much time do you spend each day on self-care?

──●──────────●──────────●──────────●──

2+ hours　　　*1 to 2 hours*　　　*less than 1 hour*　　　*no time*

What aspect of self-care are you most aware of?
- *nutrition*
- *hygiene*
- *physical fitness*
- *other_____*

What aspect of self-care are you least aware of?
- *nutrition*
- *hygiene*
- *physical fitness*
- *other_____*

Describe 5 aspects of your daily self-care routine.
1. _____
2. _____
3. _____
4. _____
5. _____

Describe an aspect of your self-care that you enjoy and look forward to.
_____
_____

Describe an aspect of self-care that you currently do not do, but would like to include.
_____
_____

How satisfied are you with your daily self-care routine?
- *completely*
- *mostly*
- *a little*
- *very little*

Warming up

Warming up should be a fundamental part of your session preparations. It needs to be as basic as charting your treatments and changing your linens. Warming up means exactly what it implies, you warm up. Your muscles and joints need to be warm *before* you start using them in order to perform at their best. Beginning your first session with cold muscles and joints will increase your chances of strain and possible injury. [1] Think of warming up as "tuning" or "priming" your body before you begin your work.

Taking yourself through a series of mobilizing exercises is an effective way to warm up. Mobilizing, also referred to as dynamic stretching, assists the body in the warming up process by increasing circulation, range of motion, flexibility and potentially preventing injury.[2] Unlike the static positions of stretching, mobilizing moves your joints through their range of motion; warming up your tissues and getting them ready for the physical activity of your work.

The concept of mobilization is very simple: you move everything around, systematically working your way through the body, repeatedly sensing and increasing your range of motion.[3] Ideally, your body should warm up slowly, reducing stiffness. Slowing moving your head around in circles, increasing the size of the circumference or swinging your hips in circles of increasing width, are just two examples of the countless mobilizing possibilities.

How you choose to warm up is for you to decide, the important thing is that you do it before you start with your first client. After your first client, presuming you don't have large breaks between sessions, your preceding sessions should be adequate to keep your muscles and joints warm. If you have a large break between clients and your muscles have cooled down, warm up again for a few moments before beginning your next session.

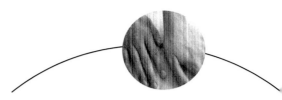

Practice tip 3.1

If you don't have a lot of time before your first session, spend just a few minutes playfully moving yourself around. Move slowly, increasing your movements as you feel comfortable. Start with your head moving down, joint by joint, to your feet or with your feet moving up to your head.

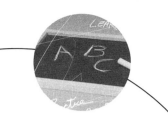

Client education tip 3.1

Remind your clients to warm up before physical activities. This is especially important for elderly clients, even if it means slowly moving their body around for a few minutes before starting their daily routine.

Self-observation 3.1

Mobilizing warm up

Begin by standing comfortably, with your feet approximately hip-width apart. Take your time and go through this exercise at a relaxed pace.

1. *Begin to move your head in circles to the left. Start by making small circles, gradually increasing their circumference. After you've made 10 circles to the left, stop and make 10 circles to the right, starting small and gradually increasing the size.*

2. *Roll your shoulders forward 10 times and then backward 10 times, gradually increasing the range of motion.*

3. *Spread your arms out to the sides and slowly circle them forward 10 times and then backward 10 times, gradually increasing the range of motion.*

4. *Circle your wrists in one direction and then the other, increasing the range of motion.*

5. *Circle your hips to the left 10 times and then to the right 10 times, increasing the circumference as you go. This is similar to the movement made when using a Hula Hoop®.*

6. *Move your entire upper body in circles of increasing width, reaching out further and further as you go. Make this movement 10 times in each direction.*

7. *Lift your left or right foot and make circles to the left 10 times and then to the right 10 times. Make the same movements with your other foot.*

8. *Slowly swing your entire body down so that your hands drop close to your feet and then swing yourself up so that your hands raise up toward the ceiling. Make this movement 10 times, increasing the swing each time.*

Resting

Resting *during* your work day is a vital part of maintaining your health and needs to be incorporated into your self-care strategy on a daily basis. Without rest, your body cannot maintain a high level of performance and will eventually become weak. It is easy to become so involved in your work that you forget to take breaks and often therapists will work through the entire day without taking a break. If you feel completely exhausted at the end of your workday, you probably are not taking enough rest breaks.

Studies have shown that supplementary rest breaks in a working regime *decrease* musculoskeletal discomfort and *increase* overall work performance.[5] Fatigue, the major side-effect of working without breaks, impairs performance quality, judgment, productivity, work efficiency, and may also lead to serious occupational injury.[6] When tired, your body cannot perform optimally and simply runs out of energy before your mind does. This causes a conflict of interests – your mind says keep going and your body says stop. Not listening to your body's need to stop increases your chance of making mistakes, putting your body at risk, as well as your client's.

During a break, take some time to rest. Even if you only have a few minutes, get into the habit of resting to help refuel, not only your body, but your mind and soul as well. Think of this time as your "recharging" time and try not to let anything or anyone interfere with it.

Taking time off from work is also important and allows your mind, body and soul to relax for longer periods of time. Everyone has different work schedules, so it's up to you to schedule time that is possible for you. For example, you might take every Saturday or Sunday just for you, spending time relaxing and rejuvenating. Schedule a day off during your workweek, or a few days every month.

The following "recharging" routine is an example of how you can relax quickly and feel rested in just a few minutes.

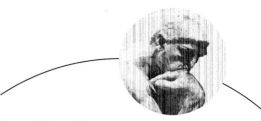

Consider this

"Current thought leans toward 'mobilizing' as being a more effective warm up than static 'stretching'. However, stretchers need not despair, mobilizing is really just a form of 'dynamic stretching' that emphasizes the motion from one position to another more than the statically held position of each stretch." [4]

Dr. Joseph E. Muscolino

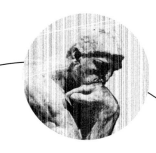

Consider this

Breathing - the ultimate rest. When you breathe, your body takes a natural rest between each time you inhale and exhale. This built-in resting point allows your body to recuperate and get ready for its next breath cycle.

Recharging

Preparation: Before you begin, you will need to find a scent that you find pleasurable and relaxing, for example, lavender, orange blossom, cedar, lemon or rosemary. You will also need something to defuse the scent. You can use a candle or electric diffuser or something as simple as putting some of the scent on a tissue and laying it near you.

It is important to use a small amount of the scent - you should be able to smell only a slight trace. You may think "more is better", but your brain needs only a very small amount to activate its olfactory center.

Begin by defusing a small amount of your chosen scent. Lie down on your table or floor. Spread your legs hip-width apart and, if you like, put a bolster underneath your knees. Allow your arms to lay comfortably by your sides. Use a small towel or pillow under your neck to support your neck muscles and, if necessary, a thin towel or pillow underneath your head.

Once you are comfortable, allow your body's weight to sink into the surface.

Bring your attention to the relaxing effects of your chosen scent.
How does the scent increase your comfort level?

Now bring your attention to your breath. (Don't change anything about how you breathe, just become more and more aware of it.)
Do you breathe slowly or quickly?
Do you breathe deeply or shallowly?
Do you breathe from your stomach, chest or both?

Now begin to slowly deepen your breath, making sure that you spend as much time exhaling as you do inhaling. Let your breath expand into your abdomen and rib cage. With each inhale, inflate your abdomen and rib cage and with each exhale, deflate them. As you breathe in, fill yourself with energy and as you breathe out, let go of any tension and stress that you may be feeling.

continued

Tip *There is a natural pause that occurs after exhaling and before inhaling. This pause helps the body prepare for the next breath cycle. Become aware of this pause as you breathe and allow it to happen naturally. It will help increase your overall relaxation.*

Begin your own natural rhythm of breathing once more and bring your awareness back to your surroundings. Slowly roll to your side and come up to a standing position. Before you begin walking, simply stand and let your body and mind adjust.

Tip *Always include the same comfortable position, pleasurable scent and breathing pattern in your "recharging" time and help yourself recharge faster.*

Self-feedback
Were you able to relax during this exercise? Explain.

_____

What element did you find most relaxing?

_____

How can you integrate a short "recharging" break into your work schedule?

_____

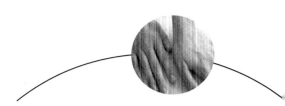

Practice tip 3.2

Here are a few ideas for winding down:

Sit quietly for a few moments. Go for a walk.

Listen to relaxing music while driving home.

Lie down for a few minutes.

Winding down

Spending time each day, "winding down" from your work life into your personal life is as important as resting. Winding down *after* your work day allows your body, mind and soul to transition from a day of work and helps prepare you for what lies ahead in your personal life.

Choose a ritual that works for you and make it part of your self-care strategy. Intentionally schedule an extra 15 minutes at the end of your day and use this time to wind down. You will be pleased with how winding down can help you more easily transition from your work life into your personal life.

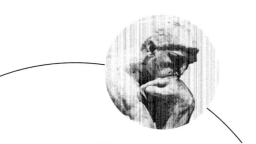

Consider this

The average adult body consists of 75% water.

Every day your body loses and must replace an average of 2½ quarts of water.

You can refill an 8-ounce glass of water approximately 15,000 times for the same cost as a six-pack of Coke™.

Got water?

Properly hydrating the body is an essential part of staying healthy and alert as a therapist. Since 75% of your body is water, it plays an important role in how your body functions. Water assists in the digestion and absorption of food, regulates your body temperature and blood circulation. It carries nutrients and oxygen to your cells, removes toxins and other wastes, as well as cushioning your joints and protecting your tissues and organs from shock and damage.[7]

Now that you know how water works for your body, let's talk about how much water you realistically need to drink every day. Experts say a non-active person should drink a half-ounce of water per pound of body weight per day.[8] For example, a person who weighs 160 pounds should drink ten 8-ounce glasses of water a day. (For every 25 pounds over ideal weight, increase it by one 8-ounce glass.) An active person, like a massage therapist, needs 2/3 ounces of water per pound. So if we use the 160-pound person as an example, he/she should drink 13 to 14 eight-ounce glasses a day.

Here are specific reasons, relevant to you as a therapist, as to why it is important to be properly hydrated:

Dehydration occurs when your body does not have enough water. When this happens, the body starts to ration available water and because the body has no reserve system, it prioritizes the distribution based on the amount available. So, for example, if you only drink 4 glasses a day, your body needs to distribute that amount carefully and evenly to each part of your body that requires water. When you become dehydrated you can experience joint, back and stomach pain, low energy, mental confusion and disorientation. For obvious reasons, as a manual therapist, you simply can't afford to become dehydrated.

Keeping your lungs moist is another important reason for drinking enough water. As your lungs take in oxygen and expel carbon dioxide, they must be kept moist by water. Your lungs lose almost 2 pints of water every day just exhaling. As we have said, breathing is a vital aspect of your self-care strategy and keeping your lungs healthy is something you can ensure by drinking enough water.

Lubrication is another reason for proper hydration. Every joint in your body is kept lubricated with water. The cartilage tissue in your joints contain water, serving as a lubricant during movement. When the cartilage is well-lubricated, your joints glide freely and friction is kept to a minimum. However, when the cartilage is dehydrated, abrasive joint friction is increased, causing joint deterioration and pain.[9] As a therapist, you need to keep your joints as healthy as possible to ensure pain-free body mechanics and a long lasting career. Proper hydration can help you do just that!

Last, but not least–your brain. Your brain tissue is 85% water and although your brain is only 1/50th of your body's weight, it uses 1/20th of its blood supply.[10] When your body is dehydrated, the level of energy generated in the brain is decreased. As mentioned, dehydration can cause mental confusion and disorientation. Many therapists experience mental fatigue, lack of concentration, headaches and a lack of focus throughout their day. Drinking enough water each day can dramatically increase your energy level, attentiveness and overall focus.

One last word on water. Many therapists say they drink plenty of "liquids" throughout their working day. But "liquids" generally mean everything else except plain water. Nothing can take the place of water, period. There are all kinds of great tasting beverages on the market, a lot of them even quite healthy. But the bottom line is this - your body needs and depends on water. And it depends on you to hydrate it properly.

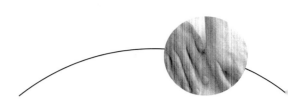

Practice tip 3.3

It's important to drink your required amount of water throughout the day, not all at once. Don't drink more than 4 glasses per hour. This will help your body, especially your bladder, to better regulate its water intake.

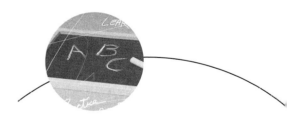

Client education tip 3.2

Remind your clients to drink plenty of water after their treatment. Water helps to move toxins and other unwanted matter out of the system. Give your clients a water bottle or cup with your business name and information on it. Not only will they be reminded to drink more water, they'll never forget where they received such good advice!

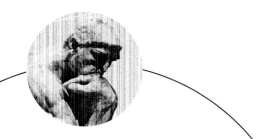

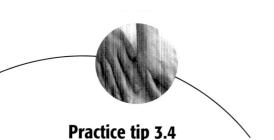

Breathing

As we have mentioned, becoming mindful of your breath and breathing pattern can aid your body, mind and soul to relax. But this is only the beginning of what your breath can do for you!

Healthy breathing is one of the most important aspects in developing effective body mechanics and preventing injuries. By healthy breathing, we mean a breathing pattern that can endure stress, and then, relatively quickly, return to normal. For example, imagine you suddenly feel pain in your back while working and your breath becomes accelerated and shallow. In this case, becoming aware of your breath and slowly bringing it back to a normal state is the healthiest approach to take. It is only after your breath slows down that you can best deal with your pain or stress. It is important that your breath supports you no matter what you are doing - talking, mentally focusing, moving around your table or simply initiating your touch. To develop a supportive breathing pattern, you need to become mindful of when your breathing is interrupted because of stress, (which is a normal response), and then allow your breathing to return to its normal state.[11]

For many reasons, remaining calm and focused during treatments can sometimes be a challenge. However, when you consciously breathe slowly and deeply, your body and mind naturally tune in to the pace of your breathing. Your body's response to your breathing pattern can be compared to your body's response to music - when you hear a piece of music that you find relaxing, your body becomes relaxed, conversely, when you hear a piece of music that is aggressive, your body becomes more stimulated. Developing an awareness of your breathing pattern will help you realize when you tend to breathe freely and when you tend to restrict your breathing. You will soon find that the quality of your breath determines the quality of your work and life in general.

Finally, a healthy breathing pattern allows your body to be less restricted, giving you more freedom to be dynamic in your body mechanics. As you have probably experienced, when your breath is restricted, your entire body becomes restricted and strained. Injuries often happen when the body is restricted in one way or another. Breathing fully and freely gives your body a sense of freedom, increasing its availability for movement and decreasing its chance of injury.

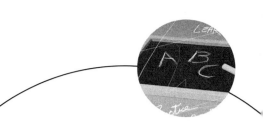

Something to think about...

Do you breathe freely or do you restrict your breathing in some way when: (if you restrict your breathing, explain why you think this happens.)

Talking with your clients?_____
_____
_____
_____
_____

Mentally focusing on a treatment area?_____
_____
_____
_____

Your body mechanics are uncomfortable?_____
_____
_____
_____

Initiating your touch?_____
_____
_____
_____

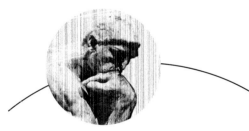

Client education tip 3.3

Lead your clients through Self-observation 3.3. Feel free to break the exercise up into parts, taking several sessions to complete it. Breathing awareness exercises, such as this one, can be very beneficial to those with chronic pain and fatigue.

Consider this

"...the quality of our breathing is the point in question, not the fact that we breathe."[12]

Carol Speads

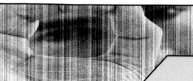

Breathing awareness

Note: Ask your partner to read this exercise to you. Also ask them to notice any changes they see in your breathing pattern from beginning to end. (Let them know that they will be asked to give you feedback regarding the changes they have noticed.)

Lie down on your table or floor. Spread your legs hip-width apart and, if you like, put a bolster underneath your knees. Allow your arms to lay comfortably by your sides. If needed. use a small towel or pillow underneath your head.

Once you are comfortable, allow yourself to feel your body's comfort.
Sense the table or floor supporting your weight.

Now bring your attention to your breath.
(Don't change anything about how you breathe, just become more and more aware of it.)
Do you breathe deeply and slowly?
Do you breathe shallowly and quickly?

Begin to notice the length of your inhaling.
Is it short or long?

Begin to count, for example, 1-2-3, the length of time it takes you to inhale once. Repeat this counting enough times so that you eventually become aware of the length of each inhale.
(Remember, at this point you are counting the length of your normal breathing pattern.)

Now slowly increase the length of your inhaling, for example, if you counted 1-2-3 in the beginning, now add one mark of time, counting to, for example, 4. (If at the beginning you noticed that your inhales were shallow and short in length, take this opportunity to breathe a bit more deeply, lengthening your count.) After a few breath cycles, add one more count of time, so that eventually you are taking long and deep inhales.

Notice your body's response to how you inhale now.
Does your body feel more relaxed and calmer?
What is your mind's response to this breathing pattern?

Rest for a moment.

Begin to notice the length of your exhaling.
Is it short or long?

Begin to count, for example, 1-2-3, the length of time it takes you to exhale once. Repeat this counting enough times so that you eventually become aware of the length of each exhale.

continued

Now slowly increase the length of your exhaling, for example, if you counted 1-2-3 in the beginning, now add one mark of time, counting to, for example, 4. (At the beginning, if you noticed that your exhales were shallow and short in length, take this opportunity to exhale a bit more fully, lengthening your count.) After a few breath cycles, add one more count of time, so that eventually you are deeply exhaling.

Notice your body's response to how you exhale now.
Does your body feel more relaxed and calmer?
What is your mind's response to this breathing pattern?

Rest again.

Now shift your attention to the natural resting point that occurs after you exhale and before you inhale. As you did with each inhale and exhale, count this resting point.

Tip The length of this resting point is different for everyone. Some people have a long resting point, others have a short one.

Continue counting your resting point, becoming familiar with its natural length.

Rest.

Now bring your attention to and count each part of your full, three-part breathing cycle: your inhale, exhale and resting point.

How has your breathing pattern changed?
Are your inhales longer and deeper?
Are your exhales longer?
Are your resting points comfortable in length?

Notice your body's response to your breathing pattern now.
Does your body feel more relaxed and calmer?
What is your mind's response to this breathing pattern?

Adapt this relaxed and calm breathing pattern to maintain your focus, remain relaxed and calm and stay centered.

Self and partner feedback
How did your breathing pattern change throughout the exercise?

_____

What differences, from beginning to end, did your partner notice?

_____

What changes do you sense in your body now, compared to the beginning of the exercise?

_____

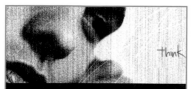

think

Something to think about...

Think about the last time you danced with someone. Was it a good experience or was it uncomfortable? Explain.

_____

_____

_____

Now think about the last time you worked with a client. How would you describe his or her rhythm and pace?

_____

_____

_____

Was there something about his/her rhythm and pace that gave you a comfortable or uneasy feeling? Explain.

_____

_____

_____

_____

_____

_____

Rhythm and pace

When dancing with a partner, you quickly discover his or her rhythm and pace. Having a similar rhythm and pace with a dance partner makes it a more pleasurable experience. Likewise, when dancing styles clash, it can be a very uncomfortable experience.

The same is true when working with a client. It is beneficial to identify a client's rhythm and pace and to work harmoniously with it. If, for example, a client is moving slowly, making quick movements around her might put her on guard. On the other hand, if a client is anxious and is moving quickly, moving slowly and calmly can help her calm down. It is also important to note that rhythm and pace can change depending on a person's emotional and physical state. Finding a constant balance between your rhythm and pace and your client's is ideal.

In the previous section, you experienced the rhythm and pace of a relaxed breathing pattern and how they can influence the overall state of body and mind. As with breathing, physical movements also have their own rhythm and pace, and it is in these elements where you find the true dynamics of your body mechanics. Whether you have a fast and syncopated movement style or a slow and steady style, it is the rhythm and pace of your body mechanics that ultimately set the tone for your individual style as a manual therapist.

While it is important that you discover the pace and rhythm of your body mechanics, it is not always simple. So, let's explore a more inherent, everyday rhythm and pace. The following exercise will help you discover your walking rhythm and pace.

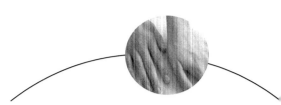

Self-observation 3.4

Walking rhythm and pace

Walk around for a few minutes in your normal manner, don't change your style.

Notice your pace. (Your pace is basically the speed at which you walk.)
Do you have a fast or slow walking pace?

Walk around until you can clearly identify your walking pace.

Now bring your attention to your walking rhythm.
What sounds can you hear in the rhythm of your walking?
Can you hear a rhythmical pattern?
What patterns of movement do you sense?

Tip There are a few ways to become aware of your walking rhythm: *Listen* for a reoccurring pattern of sound, e.g., you may hear your right foot, more than your left, hitting the floor with greater strength, sounding like a pattern of sound, a specific rhythm. *Feel* for a reoccurring pattern of movement, e.g., you may sense your right leg swinging more forward than your left leg, your left shoulder swinging more forward than your right shoulder, or your head tilting right and left. All of these sensations of movement amplify your walking rhythm and pace.

Simply walk around now and enjoy feeling your own unique style of walking.

Now that you have discovered your walking rhythm and pace, it will be easier for you to discover the rhythm and pace of your body mechanics. Because we naturally carry over movement patterns from one environment to the next, you may find your walking rhythm and pace to be very similar to your working rhythm and pace.

Self-feedback
How would you describe your walking pace?

_____

How would you describe your walking rhythm?

_____

In general, how would you describe your overall walking rhythm and pace?

_____

Practice tip 3.5

The next time you greet a client, notice the qualities of his or her movements. For example, are his/her mannerisms slow and relaxed or fast and uneven? Does he/she speak quickly or slowly? Does he/she breathe deeply or shallowly? Noting characteristics of your client's movements will help you identify his/her unique rhythm and pace.

Integrating the basics

Now that you have had an opportunity to read about and study the outside and inside basics, it is time to integrate them. Though each one stands alone as an important element in your daily practice, they all meld together. Increasing your awareness of each element while keeping an overview of their entirety will profoundly enhance your self-care strategy.

The following *Partner practice* will give you a sense of how to incorporate the basics into your daily self-care strategy.

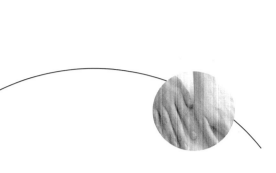

Practice tip 3.6

The next time you work, notice your own natural rhythm and pace: Do you have a slow or fast pace? Do you have a steady or syncopated rhythm? Increasing awareness of your unique rhythm and pace and acknowledging your client's will enhance your working relationship.

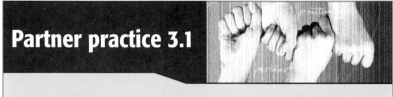

Partner practice 3.1

Building awareness of the "outside" and "inside" basics.

Begin this exercise by taking a few minutes to warm up.
If needed, refer to Self-observation 3.1.

How does your body feel now, compared to beginning a session without warming up?
Do you notice a better sense of flexibility?
Do you feel less stiff or tense?
Can you imagine warming up before each working day?

Now bring your attention to the height of your table.
Is it comfortable for you?
Do you need to adjust it before continuing on with this exercise? If so, please do.

Bring your attention now to the space around you. At this moment you might be in a classroom or your personal treatment space. Wherever you are, simply notice the space around you.
Are you comfortable in this space?
Do you have enough space around you?
Does some aspect of this space distract you?
How does this space affect your mood, attention and breathing?

Bring attention to the lighting in your space. Again, even if you are in a classroom situation, notice the lighting.
Is it adequate enough to clearly see what you are doing?
Do you have any eye strain?

continued

Notice the floor covering.
Is there an area rug distracting you?
Are you comfortable moving around on the floor?

Now bring your attention to the clothes you are wearing.
Are they comfortable?
Are they distracting you?
Is your waistline unrestricted?
If you are wearing a bra, does it allow you to move and breathe freely?

Now shift your attention to your feet.
If you are wearing shoes, are they comfortable?
Are they distracting you?
Are your feet in solid contact with the ground?

Notice your hair.
Is it distracting you?
Are you able to move freely without it falling into your face?

Now notice your nails.
How long are they?
Are they of a length that allows you to touch your partner freely, without worrying about scratching or hurting them?
Would you feel comfortable applying deep friction?

Notice your breathing.
Can you sense the three-part breathing cycle you experienced in Self-observation 3.4?
Is your breathing pattern relaxed and calm?

And finally, before you ask your partner to lie down on your table, do you have water available for yourself and your partner?

Now ask your partner to lie supine on your table.
Slowly begin to initiate your touch, but at this point keep your hands from moving on your partner.

Notice your breathing.
Was it disrupted by the initiation of your touch?

Now begin to move your hands slowly on your partner's back.

Again notice how your breathing is affected by the movement of your hands.
Can you continue to breathe in a relaxed and calm manner?

Bring your awareness now to your pace.
Do you have a slow pace?
Do you have a fast pace?

continued

Notice your rhythm.

Do you have a steady, uninterrupted rhythm?

Do you have a syncopated rhythm?

Notice if your rhythm and pace correspond with your breathing pattern.

Does your rhythm and pace match that of your breathing pattern?

Are your rhythm and pace different to that of your breathing pattern?

As you continue to move your hands, become aware of your partner's rhythm and pace.

How would you describe his or her rhythm and pace?

Notice if your rhythm and pace is compatible with that of your partner's.

If it is, how does this feel to you and your partner?

If it is not, how does this difference affect your touch?

Now purposely change your rhythm and pace so that it is very different from that of your partner's.

Notice how this change feels to you.

How does this change feel to your partner?

Once again, work compatibly with your partner. Before you stop, take a few moments, thinking through all of the elements of this exercise.

Before starting your first session of the day, take a few minutes to become aware of your outside and inside basics. If you notice aspects that are not right for you, take the time to change them. Becoming more aware of and sensitive to your environment, externally and internally, will enhance the quality of your sessions for you and your client.

Self and partner feedback

What aspects regarding yourself and/or your partner did you become aware of?

_____

How did increased awareness affect your interaction with your partner?

_____

Did you learn anything that surprised you? Explain.

_____

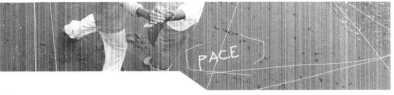

Summary

The inside basics are aspects of your internal working environment and important to keep in mind before, during and after your sessions. Here is a review:

Warming up, *before* beginning your first session, is essential to decrease the chances of strain and possible injury. **Resting** *during* your work day is a vital part of maintaining your health and needs to be incorporated into your self-care strategy on a daily basis. **Winding down** *after* your work day allows your body, mind and soul to make the transition from a day of work and helps prepare you for what lies ahead in your personal life.

Together, water and oxygen prove to be two elements we can not live without. As a manual therapist, you need to incorporate enough of both into your daily self-care strategy. Here's why: Proper **hydration** assists in the digestion and absorption of food, regulation of body temperature and blood circulation, transportation of nutrients and oxygen to cells, removal of toxins and other wastes, cushioning of joints and protection of tissues and organs. Thus, properly hydrating the body is an essential part of staying healthy and alert as a therapist.

To develop a supportive **breathing** pattern, you need to become mindful of when your breathing is interrupted because of stress and then allow your breath to return to its normal state. Healthy breathing allows your body to be more available for movement, which allows for unrestricted and effective body mechanics.

Finally, whether you have a fast and syncopated movement style or a slow and steady one, it is the **rhythm and pace** of your body mechanics that ultimately set the tone for your individual style as a manual therapist.

Now that you've read this chapter...

How would you rate your awareness of the "inside basics"?

●————————————●————————————●————————————●

always aware　　*mostly aware*　　*sometimes aware*　　*not very aware*

What part of your "inside basics" were you most aware of?
- *warming up*
- *resting and winding down*
- *breathing and hydration*
- *other_____*

What part of your "inside basics" were you least aware of?
- *warming up*
- *resting and winding down*
- *breathing and hydration*
- *other_____*

Describe 5 aspects of your "inside basics".

1. _____
2. _____
3. _____
4. _____
5. _____

Describe an aspect of your "inside basics" that you enjoy and feel comfortable with.

_____
_____

Describe an aspect of your "inside basics" which you will now pay more attention to.

_____
_____

How satisfied are you with your understanding of the "inside basics"?
- *100%*
- *75%*
- *50%*
- *25%*

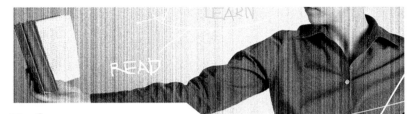

References

1.   *Exercise - Injury Prevention.* Australian Physiotherapy Association. 14 April 2003.www.betterhealth.vic.gov.au. 28 August 2003.

2.   Mackenzie, Brain. *Mobility.* Sports Coach. 20 July 2003. www.brianmac.demo n.co.uk. 28 August 2003.

3.   Ingraham, Paul. *Mobilizing: A Warm-Up Exercise Method.* www.vancouvermassage.ca/articles/exercise/mobilizing.html. 18 June 2003.

4.   Muscolino, Joseph E. *Electronic Communication.* June 2003.

5.   Taylor, Kevin. *An Overview of the Research on RSI and the Effectiveness of Breaks.* www.workplace.com. Niche Software Ltd. 2003.15 August 2003.

6.   Rohmert, V. *Problems of Determination of Rest Allowances. Part 1 & 2.* Applied Ergonomics, Vol. 2,3,4, 1973.

7.   Gallimore, Roger and Cynthia. *Importance of Drinking Water for Better Health & Weight Loss.* www.members.aol.com/savemodoe2/importance.htm 12 February 2003.

8.   *Healthy and Living Well Through Water...* www.water.com/home.asp. 17 February 2003.

9.   Sherback, Terry and Linda. *Importance of Drinking Water During the Day!* www.geocities.com/sherbs/drinking.htm 17 February 2003.

10.   *Healthy and Living Well Through Water...* www.water.com/home.asp. 17 February 2003.

11.   Speads, Carol. *Ways to Better Breathing.* Great Neck, NY: Morrow 1986.

12.   Johnson, Don Hanlon. *Bone, Breath, & Gesture: Practices of Embodiment.* Berkeley, CA: North Atlantic Books 1995.

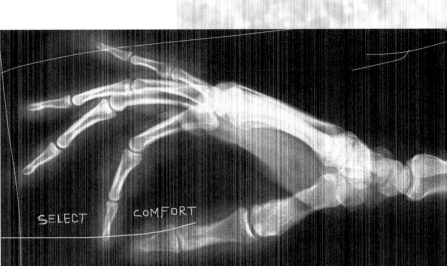

4 Tools of the Trade

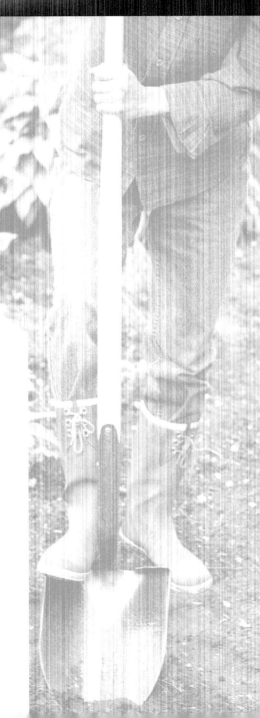

Introduction

When we talk about the "tools of the trade" we mean specific aspects of the body that you rely on to carry out your manual therapy, mainly, aspects of your hands, arms and legs. Don't be misled, however, into thinking that these aspects are the most important tools. The most important tool is your *entire* body.

Integrating your entire body, using your body's weight, proper joint alignment and a variety of movements will help develop dynamic body mechanics, ensuring the successful use of your hands. Keep these concepts in mind as you read this chapter and remember that just because we are talking about specific aspects of the hand, arm, foot and leg does not mean we are excluding the rest of the body.

Whenever possible, use your "non-working" hand to support your working hand. For example, if you are using your right thumb to apply pressure, your left hand can help support it or if you are using your left elbow to apply pressure, your right hand can help guide it across the tissue. As a general rule, two hands are better than one.

Finally, become comfortable with using both hands and arms. Typically, it is when one aspect of the hand is primarily used for work that symptoms of overuse begin. Integrating both hands and arms into your work helps to prevent symptoms of overuse and increases the dynamics of your body mechanics and treatment repertoire.

With 27 bones, 34 muscles (intrinsic and extrinsic), 40 articulating surfaces, 47 tendons and approximately 80 ligaments, the hand is a miracle of biomechanics and is said to be one of the most remarkable adaptations in the history of evolution.[1] Without fail, when the function of the hand is discussed, its prodigious capabilities for delicate and refined skills are praised. Clearly our hands have been adapted for an unlimited number of functions. However, even though our hands may seem like a "handy" all-in-one-tool, they fail "hands down" when it comes to a specific ability – the capacity to bear weight.

If we contemplate the remarkable structure of the hand, it is easy to understand why, even though the hand can perform some extraordinary manipulations, its complex and delicate structure simply cannot bear weight for long periods of time. With that said, though your work as a manual therapist is carried out using your entire body, your hands are your primary manipulative tools. At times your work requires you to use your hands in many different ways and some include bearing weight. Therefore, in this chapter we will discuss each aspect of the hand, explaining safe and effective ways to use your hands in order to ensure their health and the longevity of your practice.

Also discussed here are ways in which you can use your forearm, elbow, foot, knees and lower leg to apply pressure, and how to integrate the movement of your entire body into your work so as to better assist the function of your hands.

Before you read this chapter…

How aware are you of how you use your hands on a daily basis?

always aware   mostly aware   sometimes aware   not very aware

What parts of your hand are you most aware of?
- wrist joint and wrist
- palm and heel of the hand
- fingers and thumb
- other_____

What parts of your hand are you least aware of?
- wrist joint and wrist
- palm and heel of the hand
- fingers and thumb
- other_____

Describe 5 different parts of your hand and how you use them on a daily basis.
1. _____
2. _____
3. _____
4. _____
5. _____

Describe an everyday activity that you feel your hands perform with ease and comfort.
_____
_____

Describe an everyday activity that you feel your hands perform with difficulty or discomfort.
_____
_____

How relaxed are your hands on an everyday basis?
- always
- mostly
- sometimes
- very seldom

Your wrist joint

Repetitive movements of the wrist joint (radiocarpal joint) are found in every form of manual therapy. Whether you perform sports, clinical, relaxation or other types of therapy, you undoubtedly move your wrist joint in several different and repetitive ways. An important point to remember is that your wrist joint connects your hand and forearm, and therefore takes the stress of overuse and sustained pressure.

Ulnar deviation (adduction), radial deviation (abduction), flexion and extension are movements of the wrist joint and are used separately and in combination when performing manual therapy. When these movements are used repetitively and/or with sustained pressure, your wrist joint and the structures passing through it, from the forearm to the hand, are susceptible to injury.

Radial and ulnar deviation are frequently used in manual therapy, especially for gliding friction and when holding and manipulating a body part, for example, a leg, arm or head. (4.1, 4.2) However, movement is limited in deviation because of the structure of the wrist joint. When you use your wrist joint in radial deviation, you have approximately 15 degrees of movement and when using ulnar deviation, you have approximately 30 degrees. Furthermore, studies have shown that radial deviation causes up to a 20% reduction in hand strength and ulnar deviation, a 25% reduction. [2]

Though it is impossible to avoid wrist joint deviation, it is important that you become more aware of when and how often you use it. Whenever possible, keep your wrist joint in a neutral position to help maintain the strength of your hand and decrease the stress to the joint. (4.3, 4.4)

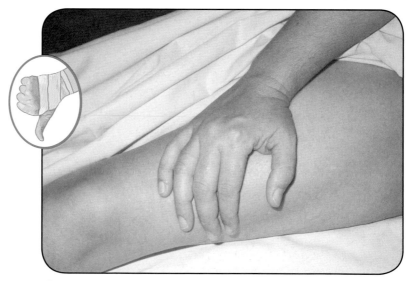

Figure 4.1

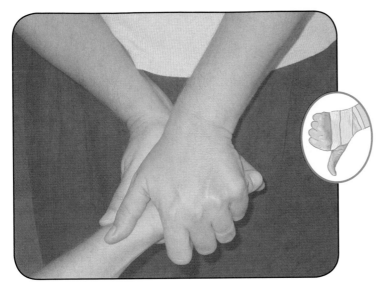

Figure 4.2

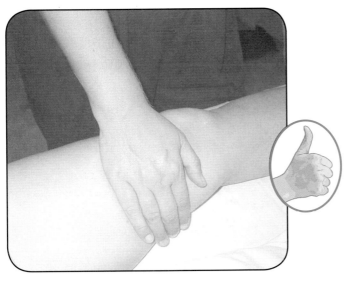

Figure 4.3

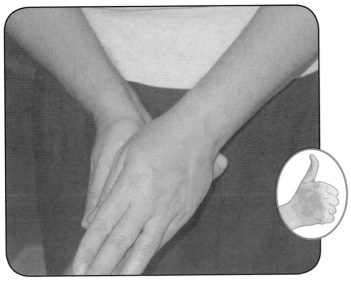

Figure 4.4

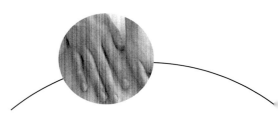

Practice tip 4.1

The next time you find your wrist joint in radial or ulnar deviation, for instance, when making long strokes down the body, try bringing your wrist joint back to a neutral position and making the same movements using more of your arms, shoulders and upper body.

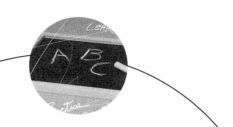

Client education tip 4.1

If your client is experiencing discomfort or pain in his or her wrist joint during certain activities, for example, when gardening or playing tennis, ask your client how she/he uses the joint. Have your client demonstrate how she/he gardens or holds a tennis racket. Notice if certain wrist joint movements are used repetitively. If so, point the movements out and see if you can find alternative movements that help relieve the stress in the joint. Simply finding a few new alternatives can make all the difference.

Flexion and extension are natural movements of the wrist joint when using the different aspects of your hand. However, holding your wrist joint in either position for long periods of time can cause instability and stress to the joint structures, especially when applying pressure. Sustained flexion of the wrist joint, especially under pressure, places stress to the joint itself and on the extensor muscles of the forearm. (4.5) Sustained extension of the wrist joint puts tremendous stress on the structures within the joint, especially the median nerve. (4.6)

To keep your wrist joint stable and safe from pain and injury, decrease the angle between your hand and forearm, especially when applying pressure and pushing. Two general rules that will be repeated throughout this chapter are: 1. Find ways to use your hand so that your wrist joint remains in a neutral and relatively aligned position with your forearm. (4.7) 2. Support your wrist joint with your other "non-working" hand and use your body weight to transfer needed pressure. (4.8)

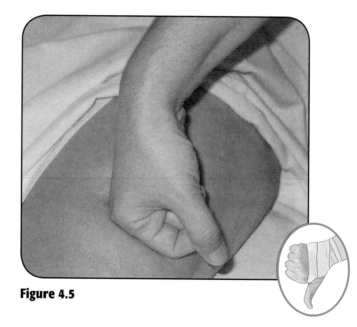

Figure 4.5

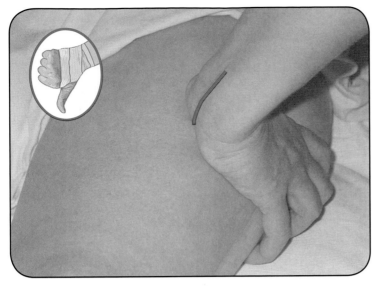

Figure 4.62 showing pathway of median nerve.

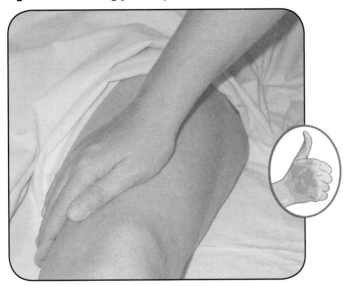

Figure 4.7

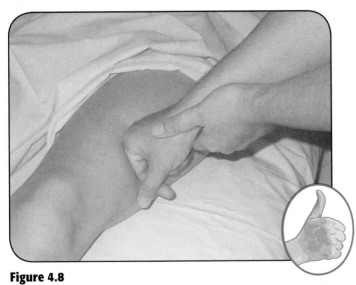

Figure 4.8

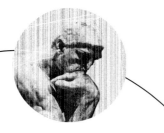

Consider this

"While the hand/wrist complex is a marvel of biomechanical engineering, the stresses that are encountered by the wrist and hand on a day to day basis by bodyworkers are tremendous. If meticulous attention is not paid to proper body mechanics, the risk of injury is great and increases over time."[3]

Dr. Joseph E. Muscolino

Something to think about...

When do you specifically use radial and/or ulnar deviation during your work?

_____

_____

Do you use radial or ulnar deviation when making long strokes down or up the body?

_____

_____

Do you deviate your wrist joint when applying deep pressure?

_____

What are some alternatives to using radial and ulnar deviation?

_____

_____

When do you use flexion and extension at the wrist joint during your work?_____

_____

_____

Which do you use more, extension or flexion?_____

Do you hold your wrist joint in extension for long periods of time? _____

_____

What are some alternatives to using wrist extension and flexion? _____

_____

_____

Your wrist

The primary aspect of the wrist used for manual therapy is the palmar side, also called the heel of the hand. Composed of eight small cube shaped bones called carpals, your wrist forms the foundation, from which all the structures of your hand pass over or through. Because of their odd shape, the carpals form bony protrusions, making them more appealing to use for pressure strokes. However, it is important to note that many of the carpal bones, by nature, are tender to the touch and can become chronically painful when pressure is repeatedly placed on them. Also keep in mind that a few of the carpals help to form tunnels that contain the two major nerves of the hand, the median and ulnar nerves. When these nerves are compressed, they press against the tunnel walls, causing potential impingement and dysfunction.

Here are more specific points to keep in mind when considering the heel of your hand for compression strokes: (4.9a & 4.9b)

The scaphoid and trapezium tubercles are tender under pressure.

The lunate, when placed under forced extension or flexion, is the most commonly dislocated carpal.

The pisiform, which protrudes from the ulnar palmar surface, can be tender to the touch, especially when used for pressure strokes.

Guyon's Canal is a small tunnel that lies between the hamate and pisiform. The ulnar nerve and artery pass through this canal. Sustained compression can cause the ulnar nerve to be pushed into the walls of the canal, causing ulnar nerve damage.[4]

The hamate has a small protuberance called the "hook" of the hamate and is tender when used for pressure strokes.

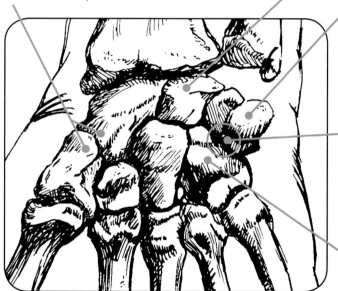

Figure 4.9a

Figure 4.9b

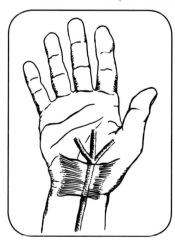

The scaphoid and trapezium tubercles, pisiform and the hook of the hamate are the attachment sites of the flexor retinaculum, the connective tissue that forms the ceiling of the carpal tunnel. The median nerve and the tendons that bend the fingers pass through the carpal tunnel. Sustained compression pushes the tendons against the walls of the carpal tunnel and may make the tendons swell, squeezing the median nerve and tendons.

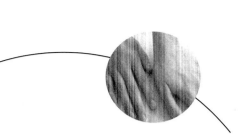

Practice tip 4.2

The next time you find yourself using the heel of your hand, for instance, when applying a compression stroke, integrate the palm of your hand into the stroke, sink your body weight into the area of focus and maintain your stability. This will take the majority of work away from the heel of your hand and disperse it throughout your body.

Does this mean you should stop using the heel of your hand? No, in fact there are techniques, such as shiatsu, that use the heel of the hand quite successfully. Furthermore, it is actually impossible to expect you to stop using any aspect of your hand completely. However, it is important that you become aware of the potential consequences of overusing your wrist for sustained pressure.

If you choose to use your wrist, decrease the stress of compression strokes by incorporating the palm of your hand to help take some of the pressure off the previously mentioned tender points and nerve passages. (4.10) Also remember, when using the heel of your hand for compression strokes, you automatically place your wrist joint in an extended position and this, as mentioned, increases instability and causes stress to the wrist joint. (4.11) Keep your wrist joint and forearm in alignment, and integrate the movement and weight of your body to increase joint stability and decrease the pressure and stress placed upon the heel of your hand.

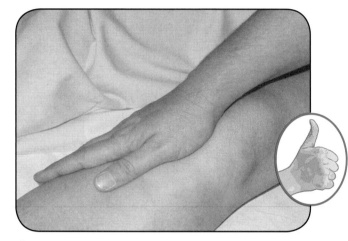

Figure 4.10

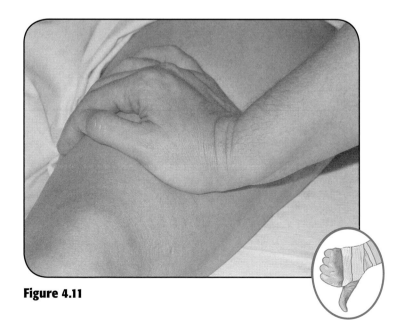

Figure 4.11

Your palm

The palm of your hand is formed by 5 long metacarpal bones, and along with your wrist, contains all 34 intrinsic and extrinsic muscles of your hand.[5] Functionally, your entire palmar surface is an effective tool for superficial and deep strokes and the palpation of energy fields. Techniques, such as polarity therapy, use the palm of the hand with great sensitivity to increase the flow of energy throughout the body. Using your palm allows you to touch a broader surface of the body with the added support of your fingers and thumb.

The advantage of using your palm is the automatic decrease of extension that occurs at the wrist joint when you naturally flatten your hand to bring your palm in contact with the body. You can add to this advantage by maintaining wrist joint and forearm alignment, and by keeping your fingers and thumb relaxed at all times. (4.12)

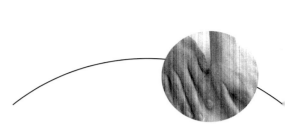

Practice tip 4.3

The next time you are giving a treatment, notice how much sensitivity your palm has compared to the heel of your hand. Can you assess the quality of the tissue, your client's breathing pattern and energy level more accurately with the palm or the heel? Is your palm more sensitive when your fingers and thumb are relaxed or held in extension? Becoming aware of the unique attributes of each aspect or "tool" of your hand can help you choose the best one for the job.

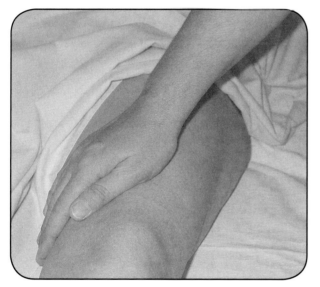

Figure 4.12

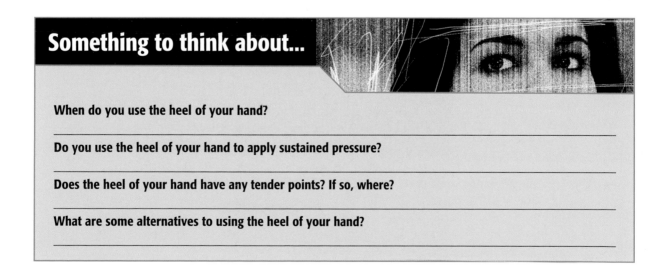

Something to think about...

When do you use the heel of your hand?

_____

Do you use the heel of your hand to apply sustained pressure?

_____

Does the heel of your hand have any tender points? If so, where?

_____

What are some alternatives to using the heel of your hand?

_____

Your fingers

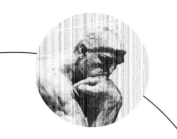

Your fingers are the celebrities of your hand. They play the most important role in allowing your hand to be the manipulative genius that it is and are the reason why your hand is a miracle of biomechanics. But all celebrities have shortcomings, don't they? Made up of 12 small slender phalangeal bones (3 per finger), 12 joints (3 per finger), and held together by only ligaments and tendons (the fingers contain no muscles), your finger's delicate structure is one reason why your hand cannot easily bear weight.

Because of their delicate and flexible nature, the fingers are best used for palpation, grasping and non-aggressive manipulations. Many manual therapy techniques successfully use the fingers for a variety of manipulations. For example, in the classic western full-body massage, the fingers are used to lift, grasp and squeeze soft tissue. The fingers are also used for friction techniques where attention to small and/or thin muscles is required. In eastern traditions, the fingers are successfully used to stimulate certain sensitive "points" on the body. Structurally, the fingers can perform many manual therapy techniques effectively if used properly and weight bearing is limited.

Your fingertips have a high concentration of nerve receptors, making them extremely sensitive. Therefore, when using them for palpation, use them gently and lightly. Once you begin to press with your fingers, you lose a certain amount of sensitivity, dulling their receptiveness.

When using your fingers for manipulations such as grasping, lifting and squeezing, keep your entire hand and arm as relaxed as possible. (4.13) Because there are no muscles in the fingers, the flexor and extensor muscles in your hand and forearm power your fingers via their tendons. When you grasp in a repetitively stiff or strained

Consider this

Palmistry (palm reading) is a method of counseling that originated in India over 3,000 years ago. It can assess an individual's character by interpreting the lines on the palm of the hand. Its roots can also be found in China, Tibet, Persia, Mesopotamia, Egypt and ancient Greece, and is still practiced today throughout the world. [6]

Something to think about...

When do you use the palm of your hand, e.g., for energy work or superficial strokes?

_____

_____

When using your palm, do your fingers and thumb rest on the client's body or are they held in extension?

_____

_____

As a client, do you prefer the touch of the palm or the heel of the hand? Explain.

_____

_____

manner, your hand and forearm tires quickly, leaving your fingers powerless. (4.14) And remember, repetitive finger movements rub the flexor tendons against the walls of the carpal tunnel and may make the tendons swell, squeezing the median nerve.

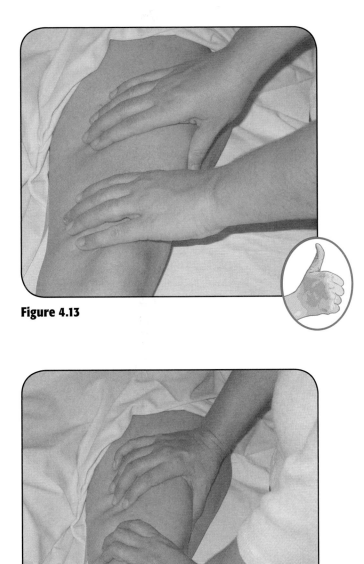

Figure 4.13

Figure 4.14

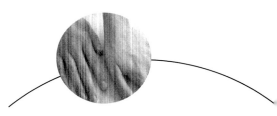

Practice tip 4.4

Your fingertips have thousands of nerve endings per square inch and are so sensitive that just one nerve ending can detect a minuscule amount of stimulation. For example, in Chinese medicine, a doctor can feel, with his fingertips, the many subtle pulses of the body. The next time you find yourself palpating the skin, take a few moments and discover how sensitive your fingertips are. Use a very light touch and explore the surface of the skin, feeling the different textures and structures. If you take a few minutes during every session, in time you will learn to use your fingertips for skillful palpation.

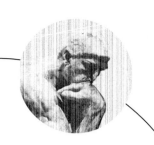

As mentioned repeatedly, your fingers are not meant for strong weight bearing manipulations. This point cannot be emphasized enough. Instead, use them for superficial friction and light pressure techniques on certain areas of the body, for example, areas that have small and/or thin muscles, including the head, face, hands and feet. When using your fingers for such techniques, do not apply pressure or friction for long sustained periods of time. Keep your fingers relaxed and, when appropriate, the joints aligned. (4.15) Pressure and stress tend to build in areas of misalignment. (4.16) Also, when appropriate, make sure your wrist, elbow and shoulder are in alignment with your fingers. The more support you can offer them, the better.

Consider this

The bones of the fingers are called phalanges because they are arranged side by side, as were the Greek soldiers in the military formation known as the phalanx.

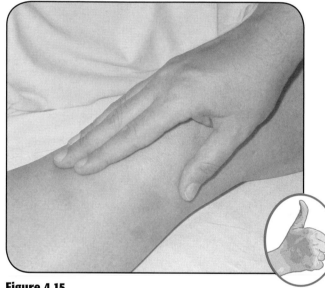

Figure 4.15

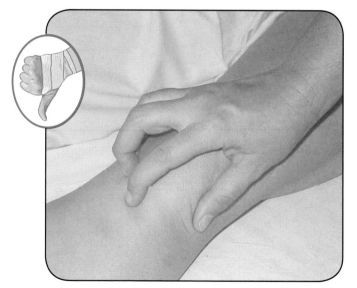

Figure 4.16

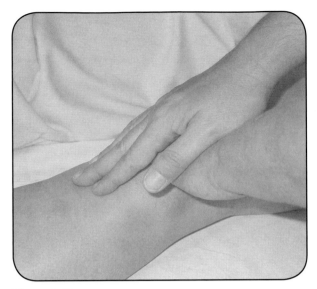

Figure 4.17

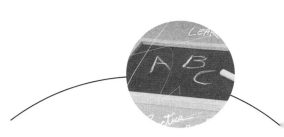

Client education tip 4.2

Often people use their hands, especially their fingers, with force and don't realize it, for example, unconsciously over-gripping the steering wheel while driving or putting unnecessary power into a hand shake. Using the fingers with too much force can potentially lead to tension in the hand, arm, shoulder and even neck and upper back. Explain this concept to your clients, helping them to understand how using less force during simple activities can decrease overall tension.

Finally, reinforce your fingers with your other hand to support them and guard against hyperextension. (4.17) It is very easy for the joints of the fingers to buckle under strong pressure, so be careful not to press too strongly with your fingers. If you require stronger pressure, choose a different tool, such as your knuckles or elbow.

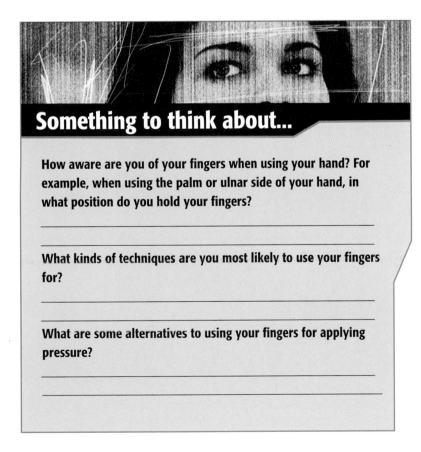

Something to think about...

How aware are you of your fingers when using your hand? For example, when using the palm or ulnar side of your hand, in what position do you hold your fingers?

_____

_____

What kinds of techniques are you most likely to use your fingers for?

_____

_____

What are some alternatives to using your fingers for applying pressure?

_____

_____

Your thumb

Your thumb has certain advantages over your fingers. Its size makes it stronger, one less interphalangeal joint makes it more stable, and its carpometacarpal joint gives it a large range of motion. It may also have a mechanical advantage of transmitting force being in alignment with the radius, the bone through which force is transmitted from the forearm to the hand.[7] These unique characteristics are perhaps the reason why the thumb is a favorite tool among many manual therapists. It is the tool of choice for techniques such as foot reflexology, where "thumb walking" is used to stimulate specific points along the sole of the foot.

Usually the thumb is chosen for applying pressure. This is appropriate if the area of focus has small and/or thin muscles or in the case where the thumb is being used in combination with other tools. Reinforce your thumb with your fingers and/or other hand when using it for applying pressure, this will help stabilize and protect its joints. (4.18) When using your thumb without reinforcement, do so for only short periods of time and make sure its joints are in alignment. (4.19) Lack of alignment can severely strain the joints and muscles of your thumb. (4.20) Keep in mind, even though it is more compact and has muscular support, overuse for strong weight bearing manipulations will put it at risk for injury.

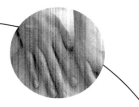

Practice tip 4.5

When performing gripping, squeezing, kneading and grasping techniques, be aware of how often your thumb and index finger come into contact and how much pressure you place between them. It has been shown that one pound of pressure between the thumb and index finger will produce 6 to 9 pounds of pressure at the carpometacarpal joint of the thumb.[8] This kind of force, on an everyday basis, could lead to joint pain.

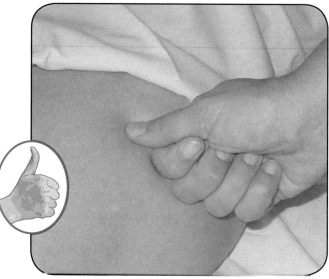

Figure 4.18

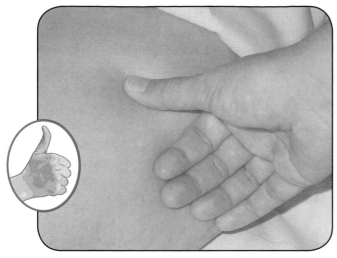

Figure 4.19

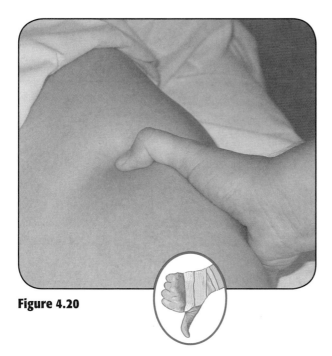

Figure 4.20

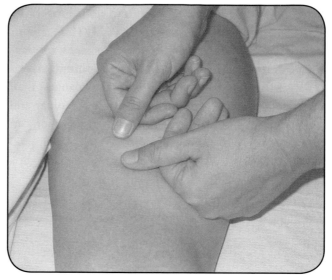

Figure 4.25

When choosing to use your fist, do not over-grip your fingers and thumb. Let them fold inward without creating undue tension in your hand and forearm. The tendency, when using the fist, is to tightly grip the fingers and thumb, often creating a "white knuckle" effect. (4.26) This tight gripping not only creates tension in the hand and forearm, but also in the upper arm, shoulder, neck and upper back.

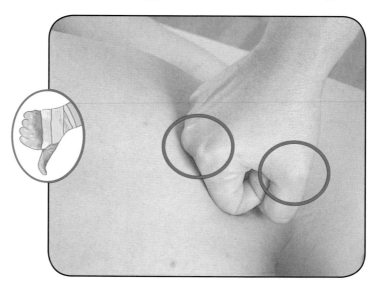
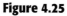

Figure 4.26

Remember to protect your wrist joint when using your fist for weight bearing manipulations by keeping it in alignment with your forearm and using your "non-working" hand for support. (4.27)

When using it to "knead" soft tissue, keep your hand relaxed.

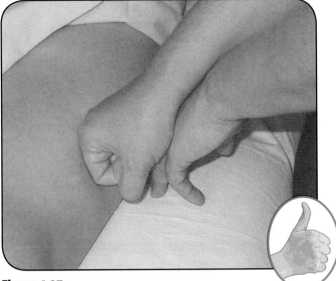

Figure 4.27

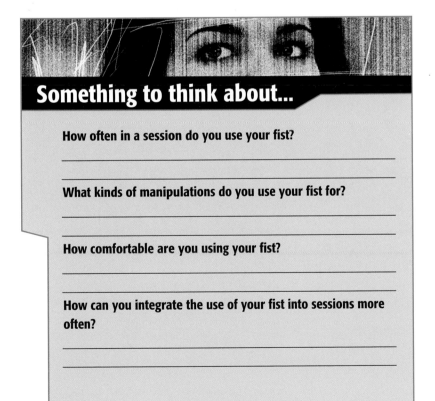

Something to think about...

How often in a session do you use your fist?
_____
_____

What kinds of manipulations do you use your fist for?
_____
_____

How comfortable are you using your fist?
_____
_____

How can you integrate the use of your fist into sessions more often?
_____
_____

Your knuckles

Your knuckles are excellent tools and nice alternatives to using the fingertips and thumb. Stronger and more stable than the fingers and thumb, when used with proper alignment, they are appropriate for light to medium weight bearing manipulations.

There are a variety of choices when considering how to use the knuckles as tools. Among them are the metacarpophalangeal joints, the "large knuckles", the interphalangeal joints, the "small knuckles", or a combination of both.

The large knuckles

Your large knuckles are appreciably more stable and stronger than your fingers and thumb, making them appropriate tools for medium weight bearing techniques. You can easily apply broad moving or static pressure by using your hand in a prone, supine or neutral position, directing your knuckles in the area of focus and using the space between your small and large knuckles for support. (4.28, 4.29, 4.30) You can use the large knuckles individually or together to create the right amount of specificity for applying pressure, both moving and static. You can also slowly rock your hand back and forth in cases where you want to apply transverse pressure with the large knuckles. (4.31)

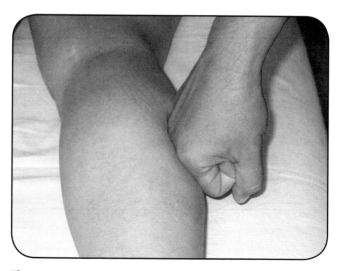

Figure 4.28

As with the use of the fist, the tendency when using the large knuckles is to over-grip the fingers and thumb, causing tension in the wrist joint and forearm. Prevent this tension by keeping your fingers and thumb relatively relaxed and, whenever possible, use the other hand for additional support.

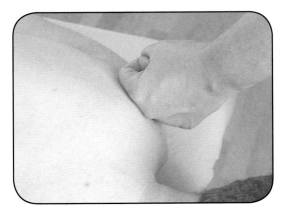

Figure 4.29

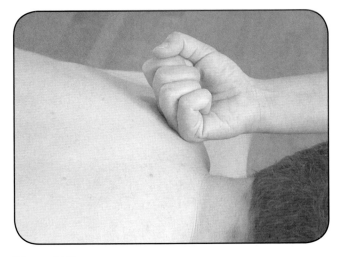

Figure 4.30

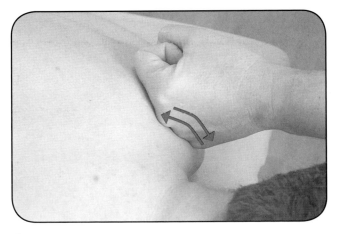

Figure 4.31

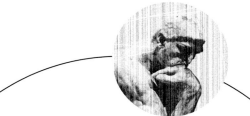

Consider this

Researchers have found fossils leading them to believe human ancestors, living three million years ago, walked on their knuckles, just as chimpanzees and gorillas still do today. [9]

The small knuckles

You naturally bend your finger to take one joint out of action when working with a small knuckle. This gives you a tool stronger and more stable than a fingertip. Because using your small knuckles gives your fingers more stability, it is appropriate to use them for light to medium weight bearing manipulations, and especially for cases where your fingertips are not adequate. They are also effective tools for any technique that your thumb can perform.

As with your large knuckles, you can apply broad moving or static pressure with the small knuckles by using your hand in a prone, supine or neutral position. (4.32, 4.33, 4.34) Like with the large knuckles, you can also use the small knuckles individually or together to create the precise tool needed for applying pressure, both moving and static.

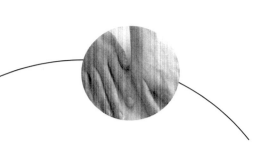

Practice tip 4.7

In eastern traditions, manual therapists use their small knuckles to knead the tissue to help stimulate circulation. Each knuckle moves, one after another, to create a "walking" effect. Try this, the next time it's appropriate, in a session. First try with one hand and then with both. Start slowly, keeping your hands relaxed.

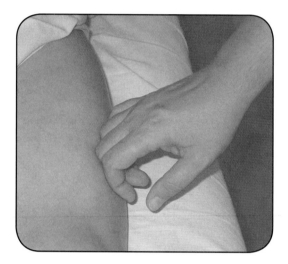

Figure 4.32

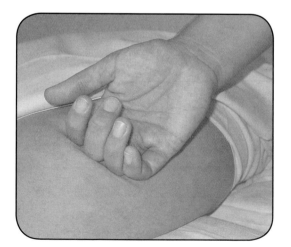

Figure 4.33

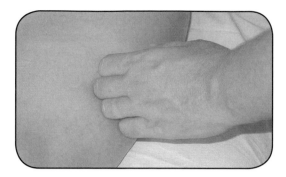

Figure 4.34

When using only one or two small knuckles, use the index and/or middle knuckle - they are the largest and most stable. Use the back of the mid and distal portion of the phalanges and the thumb to create a base of support, finding the most comfortable point where your thumb can rest. (4.35)

A common mistake, when using the thumb for support in this case, is to bring the thumb into adduction, placing stress on its carpometacarpal joint. (4.36)

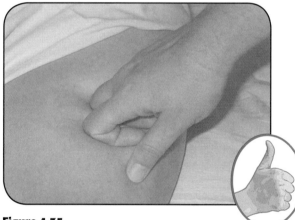

Figure 4.35

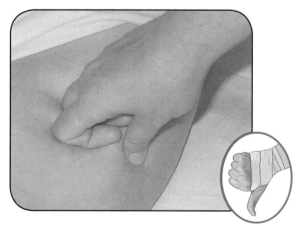

Figure 4.36

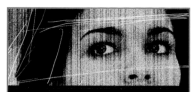

Something to think about...

What kinds of manipulations do you use your large knuckles for?

_____

_____

What kinds of manipulations do you use your small knuckles for?

_____

_____

How often in a session do you use your large and small knuckles?

_____

_____

How can you integrate your knuckles into sessions more often?

_____

_____

_____

The tendency, when using the small and/or large knuckles for applying pressure, is to flex and/or extend the wrist joint, causing stress to the posterior and anterior side of the hand and wrist joint. (4.37) Remember the general rules: Maintain wrist joint and forearm alignment and use your "non-working" hand for support. (4.38)

Finally, keep in mind that the knuckles themselves are not as sensitive as, for example, the fingers. Therefore, to avoid inadvertently hurting your client, use your other hand, whenever possible, to simultaneously palpate the tissue as you work.(4.39)

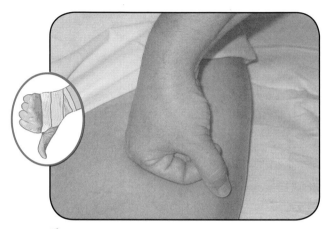

Figure 4.37

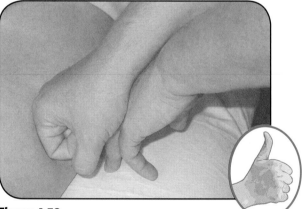

Figure 4.38

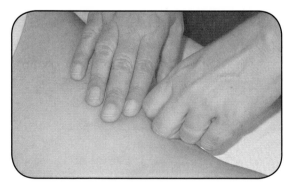

Figure 4.39

Your ulnar side

The ulnar side of your hand is relatively strong and stable, making it a very effective tool. It can apply light to medium pressure and actually manipulate tissue in the same way as your forearm, just on a smaller scale.

The ulnar side of your hand can be used for static and moving compression and kneading strokes in all positions: prone, supine and neutral. (4.40, 4.41, 4.42) Static and moving compression strokes can be done effectively on thin and thick muscles, as well as around uniquely shaped bones, for example, the scapula, clavicle and malleoli. Apply kneading strokes with the ulnar aspect anywhere you would otherwise use your fingers or fist.

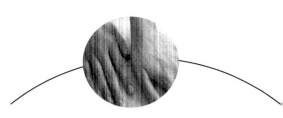

Practice tip 4.8

The next time you are working around bones, such as the scapula or clavicle, experiment with using the ulnar side of your hand to apply linear pressure to the tissue along the sides of the bone. Try using your hand in a supine, prone and neutral position to gain access to the surrounding areas. The ulnar side of the hand is an effective tool and can be integrated easily into your work.

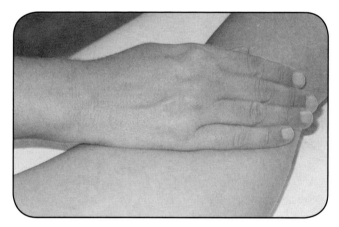

Figure 4.40

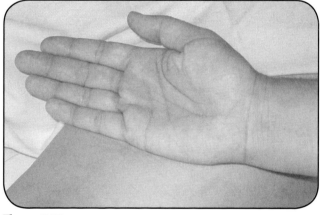

Figure 4.41

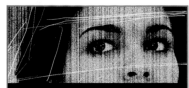

Something to think about...

How often in a session do you use the ulnar side of your hand?

_____

_____

_____

What kinds of manipulations do you use your ulnar side for?

_____

_____

_____

How can you integrate the ulnar side of your hand into sessions more often?

_____

_____

_____

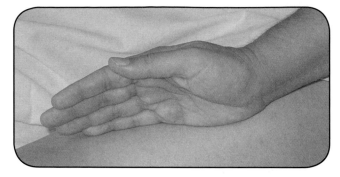

Figure 4.42

There is a tendency to deviate the wrist joint and hold the thumb stiffly when using the ulnar side of the hand. (4.43) Keep your hand in alignment with your forearm and your thumb and fingers relaxed. (4.44)

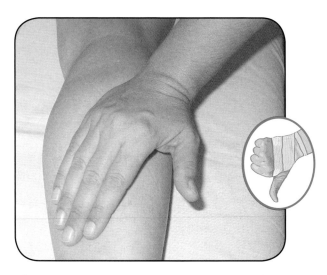

Figure 4.43

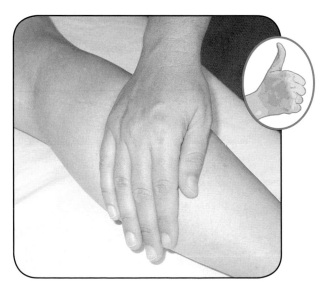

Figure 4.44

Your forearm

The area between your wrist joint and elbow, known as the forearm, is an excellent tool for applying light to heavy weight bearing manipulations. Due to its long surface, it is ideal for broad, sweeping types of strokes, increasing circulation in the area of focus faster than any other tool. Another added feature is its adaptability to all kinds of tissue. Whether the tissue is thin and small or thick and large, your forearm can effectively work with all kinds of muscle types.

The use of the forearm in manual therapy is becoming more and more common. In fact, there are some forms of bodywork which primarily use the forearm to manipulate the tissue. For example, a Hawaiian tradition of bodywork, called Lomi Lomi, uses the forearm to apply a variation of strokes to the chest, stomach, back, buttocks, legs, feet, arms and hands. This allows the therapist to cover a larger portion of the body while applying broad and deep pressure, decreasing the therapist's potential for hand and wrist joint injury.

You have a variety of surface choices when using your forearm. The ulnar side gives you a finer edge and is effective for large and thick tissue. (4.45) The anterior and posterior sides provide a softer surface and are appropriate for thin and thick tissue.

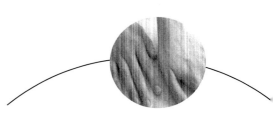

Practice tip 4.9

The next time you apply techniques with the intent to increase circulation, try using your forearms instead of your hands. Use circular or kneading movements with one or both forearms to stimulate blood flow. Remember to keep your hands and wrist joints relaxed and move your entire body to direct the movement of your forearms.

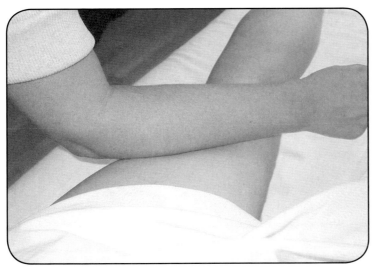

Figure 4.45

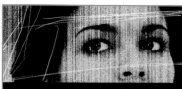
Do not hold your fingers in extension or in a tight fist. (4.50, 4.51) A relaxed hand will decrease fatigue in your hand, forearm and shoulder. And finally, transfer the weight of your body into your elbow by sinking your body weight into your area of focus and remain self-supported.

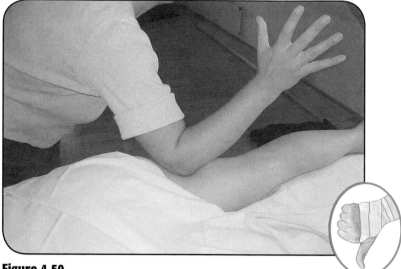

Figure 4.50

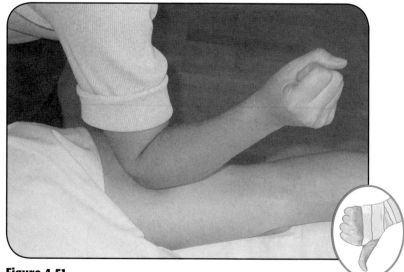

Figure 4.51

Your feet

Using the feet to perform manual therapy can be traced back to several ancient healing methods such as Thai, Ayurvedic and Chinese massage and today, using the feet is becoming more and more popular. Many therapists are realizing the advantages of using their feet and appreciating the alternative they provide to using their hands. One great advantage of using the feet is that, unlike the hands, your feet are designed to bear weight, thus using them properly to apply pressure can be done without causing stress to the joints of the feet and ankles.

If you have yet to use your feet, but would like to, start by experimenting with a willing friend. As with learning how to use your hands, forearms and elbows, learning to use your feet takes some patience and practice. Start by using one foot and as you become more comfortable, try both feet. If using both feet while standing on the body seems too unstable for you, try it while sitting on a chair.

The best way to begin is with your partner lying on a floor mat. There are some techniques where the therapist, holding on to overhead bars, works with the client on a table. However, this requires the appropriate setup. If you have the resources to create this kind of situation, try it out, but if not, start with the floor.

Make sure your nails are well-groomed and always wash your feet thoroughly before starting your work.

Like with your hands, your feet provide you with several surface options:

Use the sole of your foot to apply light to deep pressure, especially on large, thick muscles. It can also be used effectively for lengthening strokes. (4.52)

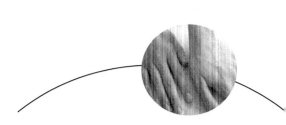

Practice tip 4.10

If you have never used your feet for manual therapy, but would like to, why not give it a try? Ask a friend to lie down on the floor and begin simply by exploring what your feet can do. Keep in mind that your foot has 40 joints and 27 bones, giving it the potential to be very flexible. Try closing your eyes and pretending that your feet are your hands, letting any hesitations go and just allowing them to move over your friend's back or leg. Begin by sitting on a chair so that you don't worry about your stability. After you become comfortable with using your feet, try standing.

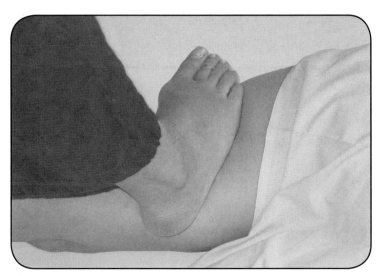

Figure 4.52

The lateral and medial sides are effective for pressure and lengthening strokes. (4.54, 4.55)

The heel, like your elbow, can be used to apply static and moving deep pressure on thick, large muscles. (4.56)

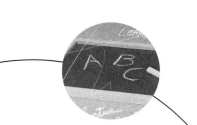

Client education tip 4.4

Many people suffer from stiffness in their feet, for instance, they have difficulty walking first thing in the morning or their feet feel stiff and sore while sitting. The next time a client is experiencing stiffness in his or her feet, show how to give a foot massage. This gives your client something pro-active to do and will most likely help to relieve the stiffness.

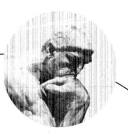

Consider this

"Although most people's feet are not as 'handy' as their hands, much of the difference lies in the lack of practice and training that the feet get for finer manipulations such as employing them for massage strokes. Given some practice, you will be amazed at how coordinated and sensitive your feet can become in time!"[10]

Dr. Joseph E. Muscolino

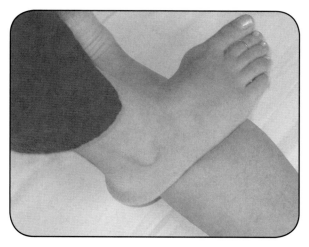

Figure 4.54

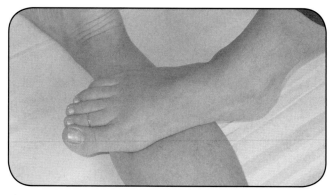

Figure 4.55

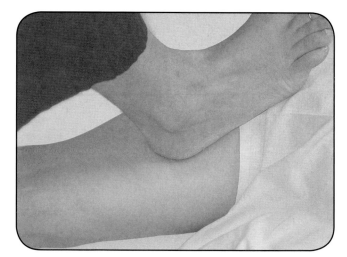

Figure 4.56

The tip of the big toe can be used effectively to apply light to medium direct pressure. (4.57) Like your thumb, the joints of the big toe cannot sustain heavy direct force through its tip. For deep pressure, use your heel.

Keep your feet relaxed and maintain proper alignment when using them. When standing, make sure your ankle and knee stay relatively aligned and remain self-supported. If necessary, use some kind of extra support, such as a hiking pole, to maintain your balance. Creating a tripod effect with your working leg, standing foot and third support piece will increase your sense of stability. (4.58)

Most of all, have fun experimenting with your feet and try out all kinds of possibilities. Your feet are wonderful tools and finding out what they can offer should be fun and playful.

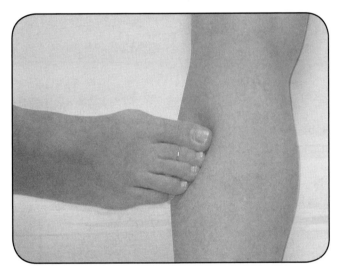

Figure 4.57

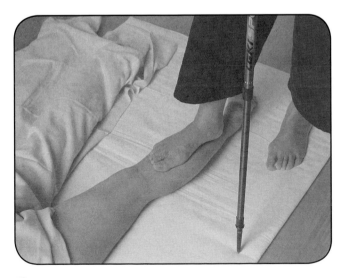

Figure 4.58

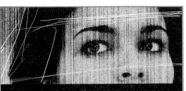

Something to think about...

Can you imagine using your feet during a session?

_____
_____
_____

If yes, how?

_____
_____
_____

If no, why not?

_____
_____

Do you have enough space in your treatment room to work on the floor?

_____
_____

How do you think your clients would respond to the suggestion of using your feet to apply manual techniques? Explain.

_____
_____
_____
_____

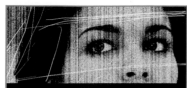

Something to think about...

When you are using your feet during a session, how could you integrate the use of your knee and lower leg?

_____

_____

_____

What kinds of manipulations can you imagine using your knee and lower leg for?

_____

_____

_____

Do you have any hesitations about using your knee and/or lower leg? If so, what are they?

_____

_____

_____

Your knee and lower leg

While experimenting with your feet, try using your knee and lower leg to apply light to deep pressure, just as you would with your elbow or forearm.

Your knee, like your elbow, is appropriate to use on large and thick muscles for both static and moving pressure. (4.60)

Like your forearm, your lower leg can be used to apply light to deep pressure and is ideal for broad, sweeping types of strokes, increasing circulation in the area of focus. (4.61)

Sink your body weight into your area of focus when using your knee or lower leg and to remain stable, use your other leg for support.

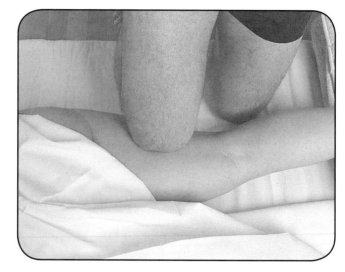

Figure 4.60

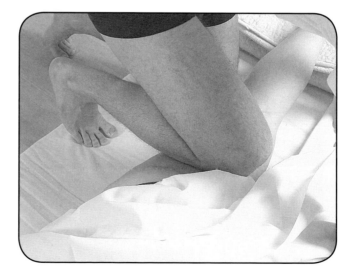

Figure 4.61

A few last words

Along with using your "tools" properly, it is important to choose the appropriate tool for both the required technique and area of focus. For example, when working with the face, you would probably choose to use your fingers. Why? Because the face has small delicate features and using your elbow just wouldn't be appropriate. But, if you wanted to apply deep pressure to the gluteals or hamstrings, which tools would be most appropriate to choose? Your fist, forearm, elbow, feet, knees and lower leg would all be appropriate choices, but not your fingers and thumb. Why not? In this case, the technique and area of focus require tools that can effectively penetrate large, thick muscles. Your elbow, for instance, can do this easily, but your fingers and thumb are too small for the job, and would be put at risk for injury. Choosing the appropriate tool for the task is the key to using your "tools" successfully.

Now that you have an idea of how to use the many aspects of your hand, arm and leg, use them - all of them. The number one reason why therapists experience pain and injury is overuse. Overuse is the result of limiting yourself to only one or two aspects of the hand for performing all manual techniques. With 78% of manual therapists experiencing job-related injuries, this is no longer a viable option. You now have many different choices and using all of them will foster your self-care and insure the health of your "tools of the trade."

Finally, use your hands and arms in coordination with the rest of your body. Integrating the movement of your entire body decreases stress in your hands, forearms and elbows, and greatly increases the effectiveness of your treatments. When the different aspects of your body are moving in synchrony with each other, for example, your lower body moving in support of your work and your upper body moving to facilitate it, your entire body moves dynamically, becoming your greatest "tool of the trade".

The following *Partner practice* gives you the opportunity to explore this concept.

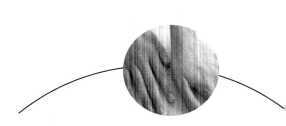

Practice tip 4.11

Explore using your knee and lower leg. Ask a friend to lie down on the floor and give it a try. You may feel more comfortable trying out the knee and lower leg than using the feet, or you may incorporate the use of the knee and lower leg with the foot techniques you have already practiced. In either case, start with the larger muscles on the back of the leg of your friend. Using your knee or lower leg, slowly sink your weight into the muscle. Experiment with applying pressure and broad, sweeping strokes.

Moving your body in synchrony

With your partner lying supine, stand by the side of your table.
Begin to move your hands up your partner's leg.

Notice how you move yourself.
Do you move only your hands and arms?
Do you move from your shoulders and back?
Do you move your upper body and keep your lower body still?
Do you place most of your weight onto your lead foot?
Are you breathing normally?

Rest.

Once again move your hands up your partner's leg, but this time only move your hands and
arms. Keep the rest of your body relatively still. **(4.62)**

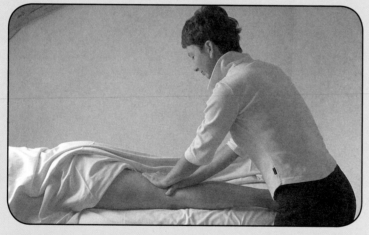

Figure 4.62

Notice how this movement strategy affects your body mechanics.
How do your shoulders and back respond?
Does this feel like a familiar way in which you move your hands and arms during your sessions?
How does this way of moving affect your breathing?

Rest.

continued

Move your hands up your partner's leg again, this time moving your hands and arms first, then moving the rest of your body in the same direction. (4.63)

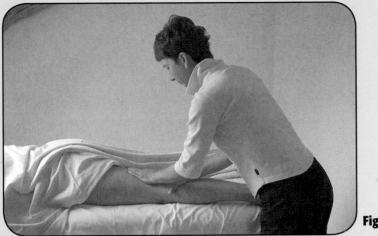

Figure 4.63

Notice how this movement strategy affects your body mechanics.
How do your shoulders and back respond to moving in this manner?
Does this feel like a familiar way in which you move during your sessions?
How does this way of moving affect your breathing?

Rest.

Now, without moving your hands and arms, move your body forward, then move your hands and arms forward. (4.64)

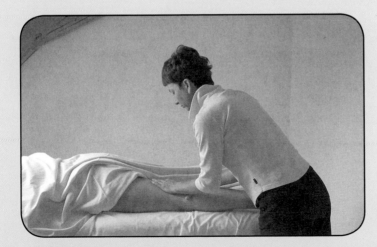

Figure 4.64

Notice how this movement strategy affects your body mechanics.
How does moving in this manner affect your shoulders and back?
Does this feel like a familiar way in which you move during your sessions?
How does this way of moving affect your breathing?

continued

Rest.

Finally, move your hands, arms and the rest of your body together as you move your hands up your partner's leg. Allow your lower body to move in support of your upper body and move your upper body to facilitate the movements of your hands and arms. (4.65)

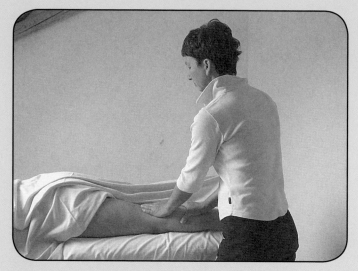

Figure 4.64

Notice how moving in this manner affects your body mechanics.
How does moving your entire body together affect your neck, shoulders and back?
Can you feel how your muscular effort has decreased?
Does this movement feel like a familiar way in which you move during your sessions?
Can you breathe more easily?
Does this feel like a more dynamic way in which to move?

Tip Transfer about 50 percent of your weight onto your lead foot and keep your rear foot in contact with the floor. If your weight cannot remain balanced between both feet, take a step up with your rear foot and then step up with your lead foot.

By dynamically using your entire body to support and facilitate the movements of your "tools of the trade", you reduce the effort in your back, neck, shoulders and hands, increase your quality of touch and effectiveness, and maintain your stability.

Partner feedback
How did moving your hands and arms in these 4 different ways affect the quality of your touch?

_____

How did it influence your effectiveness?

_____

How did it affect your stability?

_____

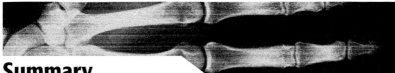

Summary

In this chapter, we have discussed each aspect of the hand, explaining safe and effective ways to use your hands in order to ensure their health and the longevity of your practice. Also discussed, were ways in which you can use your forearm, elbow, foot, knee and lower leg to apply pressure, and how to integrate the movement of your entire body into your work so as to better assist the function of your hands. Here's a review:

Integrating your **entire body**, using the body's weight, proper joint alignment and a variety of movements help to develop dynamic body mechanics, ensuring the successful use of your hands.

When the movements of your **wrist joint** are used repetitively or with sustained pressure, the joint and its structures are susceptible to injury. Support the wrist joint with the "non-working" hand and use your body's weight to transfer needed pressure.

The pisiform, hook of the hamate, scaphoid and trapezium carpals of your **wrist** are tender when placed under pressure. Sustained compression can also impinge the ulnar and median nerve.

Incorporate the **palm** of your hand to help take some of the pressure off tender points, as well as the ulnar and median nerve. Keep your wrist joint and forearm in alignment and integrate the movement and weight of your body to increase joint stability and decrease the pressure and stress placed in the heel of your hand.

Your entire **palmar surface** is an effective tool for superficial and deep strokes, and for the palpation of energy fields. The advantage of using your palm is the automatic decrease of extension that occurs at the wrist joint when you naturally flatten your hand to bring the palm in contact with the client's body.

Because of their delicate and flexible nature, your **fingers** are best used for palpation, grasping and non-aggressive manipulations. When using your fingers for manipulations such as grasping, lifting and squeezing, keep your entire hand and arm as relaxed as possible. Repetitive finger movements rub the flexor tendons against the walls of the carpal tunnel and may make the tendons swell, squeezing the median nerve. Do not apply pressure or friction for sustained periods of time with your fingers and make sure the joints of each finger are aligned and supporting each other.

Your **thumb** has certain advantages over your fingers. Its size makes it stronger, one less interphalangeal joint makes it more stable, and its carpometacarpal joint gives it a large range of motion. When using your thumb for applying pressure, reinforce it with your fingers and/or other hand. This will help stabilize and protect its joints. When using your thumb in combination with your fingers, allow it to relax.

Your **fist** is an effective tool for weight bearing and kneading types of manipulations. When using your fist for weight bearing manipulations, do not over-grip your fingers and thumb. Keep your hand in alignment with the forearm and use the "non-working" hand for support.

Your **knuckles** are excellent tools and nice alternatives to using your fingertips and thumb. Your large knuckles are appreciably stronger and more stable than your fingers and thumb, making them appropriate tools for executing deep weight bearing techniques. Using the small knuckles give your fingers more stability and are appropriate for kneading and light to medium weight bearing manipulations.

Your **ulnar side** of the hand is relatively strong and stable and can apply light to medium pressure. By using your hand in a prone, supine and neutral position, the ulnar side of your hand can be used for moving and static compression and kneading strokes. Keep your hand relaxed when using the ulnar side and, when using only one hand, use your other to reinforce and support the wrist joint.

Your **forearm** is an excellent tool for applying light to deep weight bearing manipulations. Incorporating the use of your forearm will decrease the overuse of your hand and wrist joint. Keep your wrist joint in a neutral position and your fingers and thumb relaxed.

Your **elbow** provides a strong and large bony process tool that can easily be used for light to deep weight bearing manipulations. Using the elbow dramatically decreases the overuse of your hand, especially your fingers, thumb and wrist joint. However, though it is a powerful tool, the elbow has little receptive ability. Use one elbow at a time and keep your other hand free to guide it.

Your **feet** are designed to bear weight, and therefore are a nice alternative to using your hands. The sole, heel, toes, and lateral and medial sides of your foot are all effective aspects to use. Keep your foot relaxed and maintain proper alignment. If necessary, use extra support, such as a hiking pole, to maintain balance.

Your **knee** is appropriate to use on large and thick muscles for both static and moving pressure, and your **lower leg** can be used to apply light to deep pressure and is ideal for broad, sweeping strokes. When using either your knee or lower leg, sink your body's weight into the area of focus, using your other leg for support. It is important to remain self-supported.

By dynamically using your entire body to support and facilitate the movements of your "tools of the trade", you reduce the effort in your back, neck, shoulders and hands, increase your quality of touch and effectiveness, and maintain your stability.

SUPPORT

Now that you've read this chapter...

How aware are you now of how you use your hands while working?

●————————————●————————————●————————————●

always aware　　　　*mostly aware*　　　　*sometimes aware*　　　　*not very aware*

What parts of your hand are you now more aware of?
- *wrist joint and wrist*
- *palm and heel of the hand*
- *fingers and thumb*
- *other_____*

What parts of your hand are you still not so aware of?
- *wrist joint and wrist*
- *palm and heel of the hand*
- *fingers and thumb*
- *other_____*

Describe 5 "tools of the trade" that you like to use and why.

1. _____

2. _____

3. _____

4. _____

5. _____

Describe your experience of using your feet, knees and lower legs.

_____

_____

Describe the aspects of your hand or lower body that you still need a little practice using.

_____

_____

How many new "tools of the trade" have you discovered?
- *1*
- *2*
- *3*
- *4+*

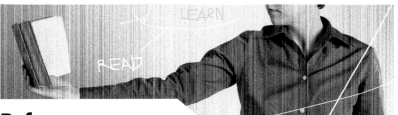

References

1. Muscolino, Joe E. *Electronic Communication.* June 2003.

2. Li Zm. *Wrist Position Determines Force of Individuals Fingers.* Biomechanics. 2002. www.vistalab.com. 31 March 2003.

3. Muscolino, Joe E. *Electronic Communication.* June 2003.

4. Swailes, Nathan. *Guyon's Canal.* Human Biology, School of Biomedical Sciences, The University of Leeds. April 2000, www.bms.leeds.ac.uk. 4 June 2003.

5. Muscolino, Joe E. *The Muscular System Manual: The Skeletal Muscles of the Human Body.* Redding: JEM Publications, 2002.

6. Palmistry. *Britannica Ready Reference.* Encyclopedia Britannica, Inc. 2001.

7. Muscolino, Joe E. *Electronic Communication.* June 2003.

8. Greider, Jack L. *Surgery of the Hand and Upper Extremity.* Southeastern Hand Center www.handsurgery.com. 17 April 2000.

9. Associated Press. *Study: Human Ancestors had Knuckle-Walking Characteristics.* www.cnn.com/2000/nature. 28 April 2000.

10. Muscolino, Joe E. *Electronic Communication.* June 2003.

5 Standing

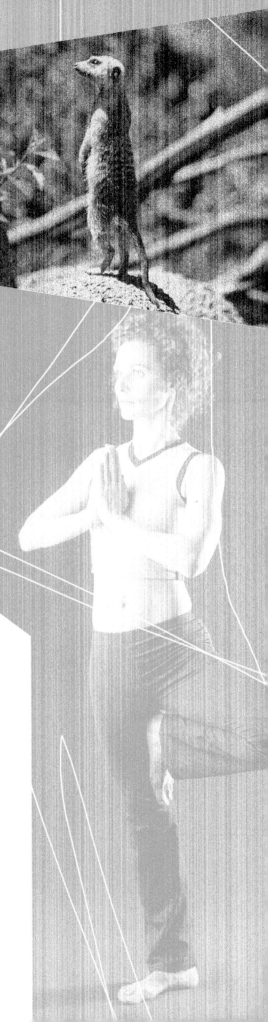

Introduction

Standing can be defined, for our purpose, as a basic functional posture from which all other body mechanics can be performed, for example, lifting, bending, pushing, pulling and applying pressure. As a manual therapist, you stand *and* move simultaneously in different ways, performing the specific techniques of your therapy. When standing is comfortable and stable, dynamic movement is possible, enabling you to effectively execute the specific functions of manual therapy. On the other hand, when standing is uncomfortable, movement is limited and execution often ineffective.

In this chapter, you will explore how to stand supported by your musculoskeletal system. You will learn how to use the "tripods" of your feet, find an effective stance, vertically balance your upper body over your lower body and your head over your spine. Ultimately, you will learn how to stand in such a way that allows you to move dynamically and effectively.

Before you read this chapter...

How often do you stand on a daily basis?

○ *almost always*
○ *sometimes*
○ *not very often*
○ *other_____*

What parts of your body are you most aware of when standing?

○ *neck and shoulders*
○ *arms and hands*
○ *lower back and feet*
○ *other_____*

What parts of your body are you least aware of when standing?

○ *neck and shoulders*
○ *arms and hands*
○ *lower back and feet*
○ *other_____*

Describe 5 standing habits you are aware of on a daily basis.

(e.g., do you usually stand on one foot or both or do you stand with weight on one hip or both?)

1. _____
2. _____
3. _____
4. _____
5. _____

Describe an everyday activity involving standing that you do with ease and comfort.

_____

_____

Describe an everyday activity involving standing that you do with difficulty or discomfort.

_____

_____

How comfortable are you standing on an everyday basis?

○ *always*
○ *mostly*
○ *sometimes*
○ *very seldom*

Balanced Standing

Standing is a basic functional posture of manual therapy. Whether you stand for a short period of time or the entire length of your session, standing is a requirement of your work. You may find yourself standing quietly during your sessions, or moving from one position to the next, performing a variety of techniques, such as applying pressure. No matter what role standing plays in your sessions, it is an inherent part of your body mechanics. Therefore, it is prudent that you learn how to stand using the support of your musculoskeletal system, with a balance between stability and a readiness for movement. (5.1)

Though it may seem relatively simple, finding a stable and comfortable standing position can be a difficult task. Most people try to stand "still" and/or "straight" in their endeavor to find stability and comfort, but end up feeling even more uncomfortable in the process. Why? The fact is, the body must continue to move or "sway" in varying degrees in order to keep itself balanced and in-check with gravity.[1] Trying to stand "still" only creates a reflex for your body to move more. Trying to stand "straight" is also futile, yet it is common to see people attempting to stand "straight", with their shoulders back, chins up and knees locked. (5.2) Your mother or teacher might have

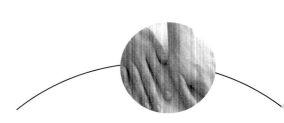

Practice tip 5.1

When standing, therapists become so involved with their work that they forget to move - even breathe. When you are working, do not allow yourself to remain in a fixed or static position. Remember, you are always free to move, no matter how intense your session may be. Find a picture that depicts dynamic movement and put it in your treatment room. When you sense yourself standing in a static manner, take a look at the picture. It will help bring the sense of movement back into your body.

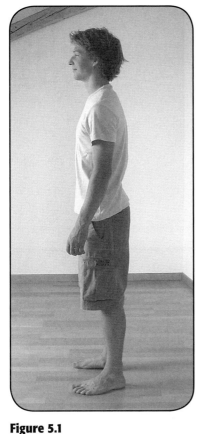

Figure 5.1

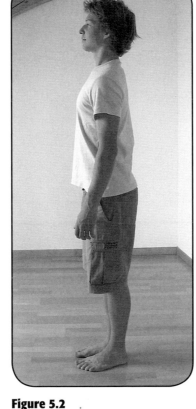

Figure 5.2

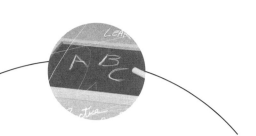

Client education tip 5.1

Often people do not realize how they stand. If you have a client with the tendency to stand "straight", show him/her the shape of the skeleton, explaining how its curves are required for movement. Suggesting a more relaxed posture can help make standing a more pleasurable experience.

told you to "stand up straight" with the hopes of improving your posture, but the truth is, standing "straight" takes your skeleton out of its natural curvature and requires your muscles to work hard to hold a "straight" and static posture.

So, how do you find a balanced standing posture? Your musculoskeletal system holds all the keys and we will discuss each of them throughout the rest of this chapter. By utilizing the "tripods" of your feet, finding a stable stance, vertically aligning your upper and lower body and your head over your spine, your standing posture will be stable and comfortable, enabling you to move from one position to the next, effectively.

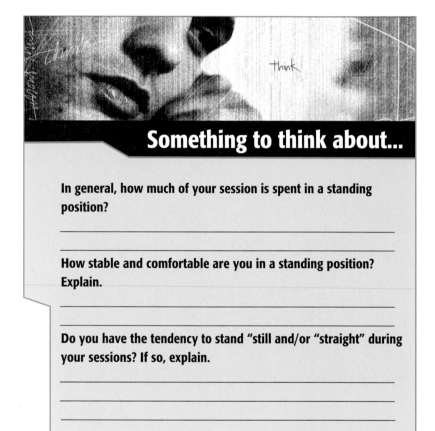

Something to think about...

In general, how much of your session is spent in a standing position?

_____

_____

How stable and comfortable are you in a standing position? Explain.

_____

_____

Do you have the tendency to stand "still and/or "straight" during your sessions? If so, explain.

_____

_____

_____

Standing on your "tripods"

When standing, walking or running, your feet bear the weight of your entire body. In fact, during a typical day, they endure a cumulative force of several hundred tons.[2] It is not difficult to understand why many therapists complain of sore and tired feet at the end of a long day's work. Standing in a balanced manner starts with learning how to use your feet effectively and dynamically.

To begin, it is helpful to understand the general structure of your foot. It contains 26 bones, 40 joints, 38 muscles and a network of more than 100 tendons, ligaments, blood vessels and nerves.[3] With regard to standing, many of the structures in your foot are arranged to form arches that work together, raising the center of your foot, creating a "bridge" of support. (5.3)

This bridge acts to distribute and absorb the weight of your body. This is extraordinary considering how relatively small the feet are!

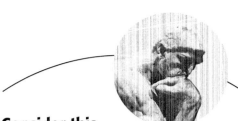

Consider this

If you look at the human skeleton, you will find 206 bones with many shapes - long, short, flat and irregular, but you will not find one "straight" bone. Your skeleton has several curves and shapes that, with the help of your muscles, give you dynamic movement, balance, shape and form.

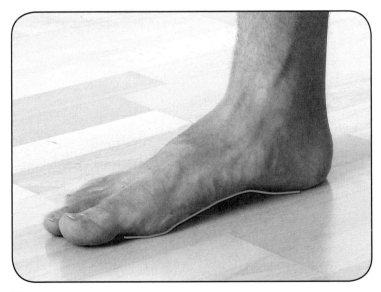

Figure 5.3

To use your feet effectively, you must employ the three points of contact formed by the three arches. They are the calcaneus (your heel), the head of the first metatarsal (base of your big toe) and the head of the fifth metatarsal (base of your little toe).[4] (5.4) Together these points form a triangle or "tripod" and, when properly utilized, can support, distribute and absorb your body's weight. When you become more aware of these three points and begin engaging them, your foot will function in a more dynamic way, making it possible to stand in a balanced manner, without experiencing undue foot fatigue.

The following *Self-observation* lesson will give you the opportunity to experience standing on the "tripods" of your feet.

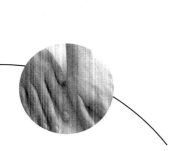

Practice tip 5.2

Are your feet sore at the end of the day? If so, try distributing your weight equally over the "tripods" of your feet. At first, making this adjustment might take some time, but you may soon find that standing on the tripods of your feet relieves foot fatigue.

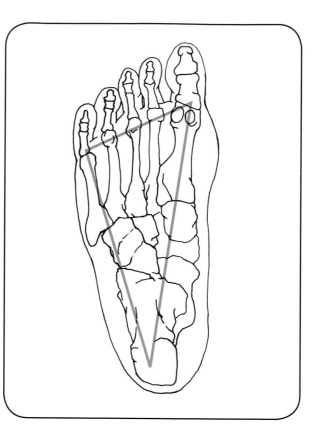

Figure 5.4

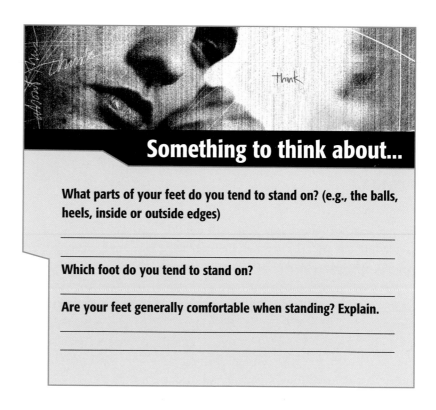

Something to think about...

What parts of your feet do you tend to stand on? (e.g., the balls, heels, inside or outside edges)

_____

_____

Which foot do you tend to stand on?

_____

Are your feet generally comfortable when standing? Explain.

_____

_____

Standing on your tripods

Take off your shoes and stand with your feet under your pelvis. Distribute your weight equally between both feet. Look down between your feet and notice the distance each foot is from your center line.

Tip Your center line is a line that, if drawn from your head down between your feet, would divide your body into equal halves.

Place your feet at equal distances from your center line. This will create a strong angle of support from which your legs can transmit your weight equally to your feet. (5.5)

Notice and sense which parts of your feet you are standing on.
Are you standing with your weight equally placed on your feet?
Are you standing more on your heels?
Are you standing more on your forefoot?
Are you standing more on the inside or outside edges?

Lean your body back so that you stand primarily on your heels. This will enable you to place weight on the back point of your foot's tripod, the calcaneus. (5.6)

Notice how standing on your heels affects your lower body.
Do you feel the muscles in your legs working to hold your balance?
Can you sense something happening in your knees?
Can you sense something happening in your ankles?
Is this a position you normally stand in?

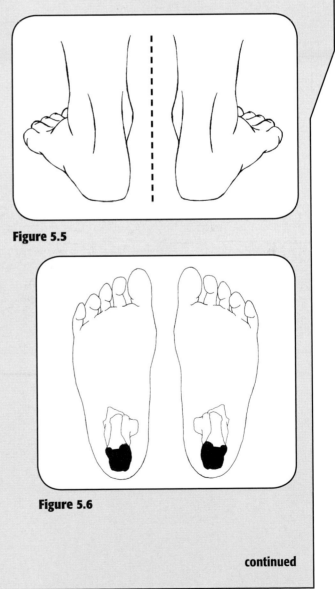

Figure 5.5

Figure 5.6

continued

Notice how this position affects your upper body.
Do you sense the muscles in your back working to hold your balance?
Are the muscles in your neck and shoulders working to hold your balance?
How does this position affect your breathing?

Rest.

Stand again and place your feet at equal distances from your center line, distributing your weight equally between both feet. Slowly lean your body forward and stand primarily on the forefoot of each foot. This will enable you to place weight on the two forward points of your foot's tripod. (5.7)

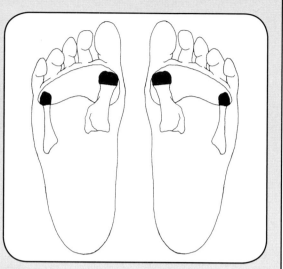

Figure 5.7

Tip A line drawn across the two forward points of your foot's tripod, the base of the small toe and the base of the big toe, would span the width of your forefoot.

Notice how standing on the balls of your feet affects your lower body.
How do the muscles in your legs respond?
Can you sense your calves working hard to keep you from falling forward?
How are your knees and ankles responding to this position?
Is this a position you normally stand in?

Notice how standing in this position affects your upper body.
Do you sense the muscles in your back working to hold your balance?
Are the muscles in your neck and shoulders working to hold your balance?
How does this position affect your breathing?

Rest.

Stand again and place your feet at equal distances from your center line, distributing your weight equally between both feet. Let your body weight travel down the strong angle formed by your legs and onto the supportive tripods of your feet. Your weight will now be supported by the heel and the width of the forefoot on both feet. Stand for a few minutes, sensing and visualizing the tripods of your feet. (5.8)

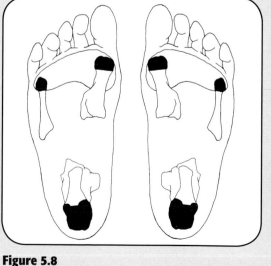

Figure 5.8

continued

Notice how standing on the tripods of your feet affects your entire body.
Has the muscular effort in your legs decreased?
Has the stability increased in your knees and ankles?
Is your back more comfortable?
Are your neck and shoulders more comfortable?
Can you breathe more freely?

Take a few minutes and continue standing on your tripods. Sense your overall balance and support.

When standing with your body's weight evenly placed through your foot's natural tripod and with your legs in a strong angle of support, your entire skeleton has a solid base on which to stand. The muscular effort of your lower body is decreased as is the stress on your knees and ankles.

Self-feedback
What was your overall feeling of support when standing on the tripods of your feet?

_____

What are the advantages of standing on the tripods of your feet?

_____

How did standing on the tripods of your feet affect your sense of overall comfort?

_____

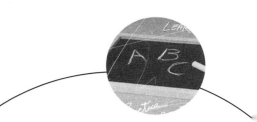

Client education tip 5.2

Sometimes, out of habit or as a result of an injury, people stand on the inside, outside, the forefoot or the heel of the foot. If a client is experiencing difficulty standing on his or her feet, show and explain the concept of the "tripod" and if appropriate, gently lead him or her through Self-observation 5.1. It will help your client gain a better understanding of the foot's structure and perhaps even alleviate discomfort.

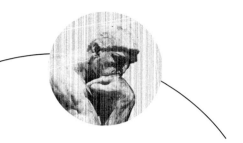

Taking a stance

Now that you have an idea of how to use your feet in a stable and comfortable manner, let's take a look at the stances used by manual therapists. Generally, there are two stances utilized by therapists. One is a parallel stance where both feet are placed side-by-side. The other is a one-foot forward stance where one foot is in front of the other. The parallel stance is usually used when the therapist is facing across the table or standing at the head or foot. The one-foot forward stance is used when the therapist is advancing along the side of the table and also when standing at the head or foot. Both stances are effective, but certain points must be kept in mind to ensure optimal effectiveness.

Forming a "T" with the feet is often a mistake made by therapists when using a one-foot forward stance. Though a "T" stance may seem like a stable position, it creates a rotation or twist in the therapist's body. While trying to direct the movement of his body forward with the lead foot, the therapist's body is turned away from the direction of focus by the rear foot. (5.9) Working with your feet in this kind of stance causes stress to the entire body, putting it in direct conflict with itself. Often, it is the low back, knee and ankle of the rear foot where most of the stress is felt. (5.10) Though the "T" stance is appropriate for such disciplines as Tai Chi, where movement in several directions is required, it is inappropriate for the body mechanics of manual therapists.

Find a stable one-foot forward stance where both feet are pointed, as much as possible, toward your direction of movement. This will not only decrease the risk of strain to your back, knees and ankles, but your body will be able to move without conflict, increasing your mobility and comfort. (5.11)

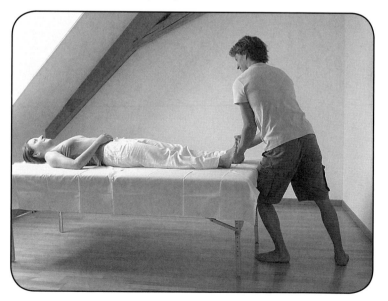

Figure 5.9

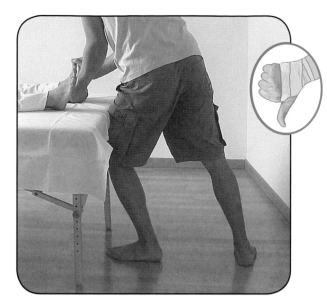

Figure 5.10

Keep both feet comfortably aligned forward when using the parallel stance. (5.12) This means that your feet are not too internally or externally rotated. With extreme rotation comes the feeling of tightness and sometimes spasm in the low back and hip rotators. If you were to hold a skeleton up, so that its feet were not touching the ground, you would see that the feet externally rotate only 15 -20 degrees. This is the natural rotation of the foot, due to the structure of the leg and its connection to the hip joint.[5] In both stances, working with the feet comfortably directed forward allows the tripods of your feet to be engaged and your lower body to support and move in a more dynamic way.

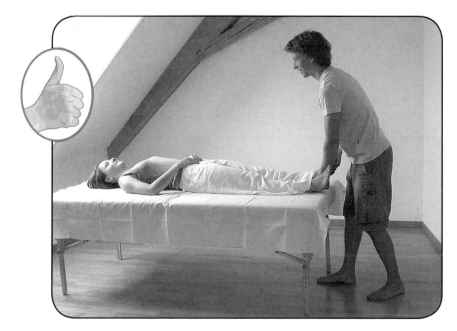

Figure 5.11

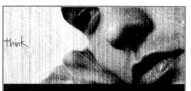

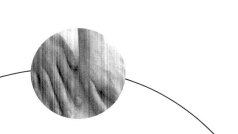

Practice tip 5.3

The next time you are using a one-foot forward stance, notice where you place your feet. If you place them in a "T", notice how this feels in your low back, knees and ankles. Notice if you can feel yourself being pulled in the two directions that your feet are pointing. On the other hand, if you point your feet in the same direction, notice how this feels in your low back, knees and ankles. Becoming more aware of where you place your feet when working leads to a better understanding of your overall standing dynamics.

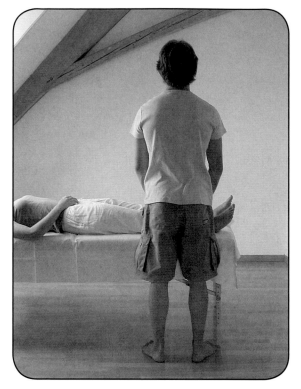

Figure 5.12

Whether you stand with your feet parallel to each other or with one foot forward, your stance should ideally transmit the weight of your body evenly down to your feet. In this situation, your legs form a triangle with the floor, putting your legs at equal distances from your center line. (Remember your center line is a line that, if drawn from your head down between your feet, would divide your body into equal halves.) With your weight evenly distributed between your feet, you can engage the tripods of your feet, increasing the overall stability of your stance. (5.13, 5.14)

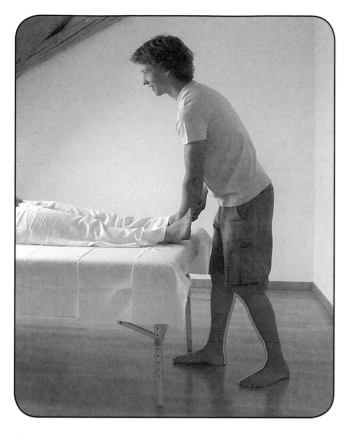

Figure 5.13

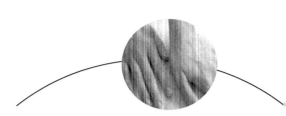

Practice tip 5.4

When you feel uncomfortable standing during a session, take a few minutes and imagine that you have a string attached to the top of your head, gently lengthening your spine. This will help increase your vertical alignment and overall comfort. Remember, don't think of yourself as standing "straight", rather think of the string as encouraging your spine to remain vertical but also allowing it to keep its natural curvature.

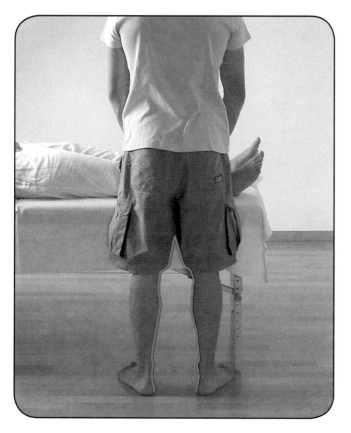

Figure 5.14

Standing vertically aligned

Now that you have learned how to find a stable and effective stance, it is time to learn how to vertically align your body. When standing, it is important to keep your upper body vertical and balanced over your pelvis, legs and feet. When vertical, the force of gravity is distributed throughout your entire body, allowing all the joints in your body to effortlessly support you.[6] Thus, no one structure is over-stressed. (5.15)

With vertical alignment, your body weight is balanced over your spine and lower extremity joints, requiring little muscular effort. However, when your body moves out of vertical alignment, for example, when you bend forward, the force of gravity is no longer evenly distributed. This increases the stress and strain on the joints and muscles of your body. (5.16) Keep your center of gravity over your feet and allow your upper body to move without restriction. Your spine, shoulders, arms and hands will work more efficiently with less fatigue and strain, moving more freely. (5.17)

To best experience the concept of balanced standing, you will be asked to stand and perform simple movements in the following *Self-observation* lesson.

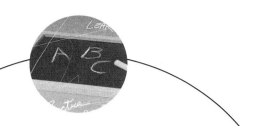

Client education tip 5.3

If you have a client with back pain, notice if he/she has the propensity to lean the upper body forward or backward from the legs. Often this pattern can put enormous strain on the lower back, causing discomfort. Bring attention to this pattern and help to find a more comfortable vertical alignment to assist your client in decreasing pain and discomfort.

Consider this

"When one body part is positioned above the body part below, it requires no effort and places no strain upon the body to maintain the position. If, however, an upper body part deviates from this vertical alignment, undue stress is placed upon the tissues of the body affecting the ease and fluidity of your bodywork." [7]

Dr. Joseph E. Muscolino

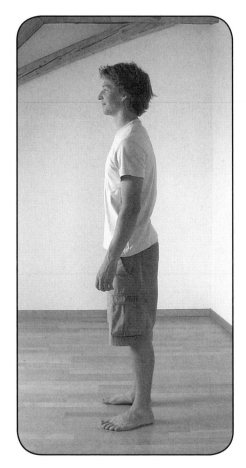

Figure 5.15

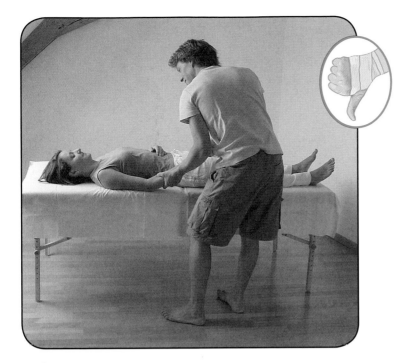

Figure 5.16

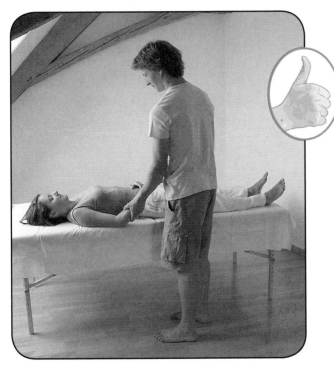

Figure 5.17

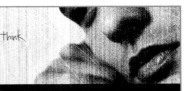

Something to think about...

When standing, where do you perceive your upper body to be in relation to your lower body? (e.g., is your upper body in front or in back of your pelvis and legs?)

_____

_____

What is your perception of the shape of your spine when standing?

_____

_____

What are the advantages of standing vertically aligned?

_____

_____

How can the concept of standing vertically aligned help improve your body mechanics in general?

_____

_____

_____

Standing   123

Standing vertically aligned

Stand with your feet under your pelvis, distributing your weight equally between both feet. Begin to bend your upper body forward, forming a convex shape with your spine. (5.18)

Notice how this position affects your balance and skeletal support.
Do you have a sense of balance in this position?
Do you feel supported by your skeleton?
Are you able to maintain contact with the tripods of your feet?
Is your weight more on the balls or the heels of your feet?

Notice how the muscles in your upper body respond to this position.
Do you sense muscular effort in your neck and shoulders?
Do you sense effort in your upper or lower back?

Notice how the muscles in your lower body respond to this position.
Do you sense muscular effort in your upper legs?
Do you sense effort in your lower legs and feet?

Notice your breathing.
Can you breathe comfortably in this position?

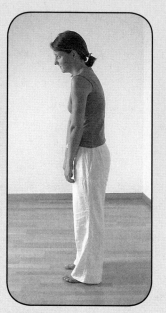

Figure 5.18

Remain in this position and slowly lift your arms out in front of yourself, as if you were going to begin working with a client.

Notice how lifting your arms in this position affects the muscles in your upper body.
Is there muscular effort in your neck and shoulders?
Do you sense effort in your upper or lower back?
Is it comfortable lifting your arms from this standing position?

Rest.

Once again, stand with your feet under your pelvis, distributing your weight equally between both feet. This time, begin to bend your upper body backward, forming a concave shape with your spine. (5.19)

Notice how this position affects your balance and skeletal support.
Do you have a sense of balance in this position?
Do you feel supported by your skeleton?
Are you able to maintain contact with the tripods of your feet?
Is your weight more on the balls or the heels of your feet?

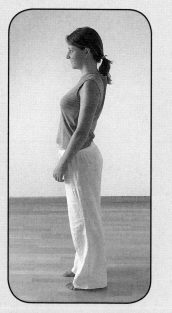

Figure 5.19

continued

Notice how the muscles in your upper body respond to this position.
Do you sense muscular effort in your neck and shoulders?
Do you sense effort in your upper or lower back?

Notice how the muscles in your lower body respond to this position.
Do you sense muscular effort in your upper legs?
Do you sense effort in your lower legs and feet?

Notice your breathing.
Can you breathe comfortably in this position?

Remain in this position and slowly lift your arms, as before.

Notice how lifting your arms in this position affects the muscles in your upper body.
Is there muscular effort in your neck and shoulders?
Do you sense effort in your upper or lower back?
Is it comfortable lifting your arms from this standing position?

Rest.

Again, stand with your feet under your pelvis, distributing your weight equally between both feet. Begin to slowly side-bend your upper body to the left. (5.20)

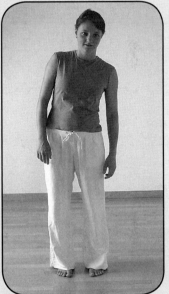

Figure 5.20

Notice how this position affects your balance and skeletal support.
Do you have a sense of balance in this position?
Do you feel supported by your skeleton?
Are you able to maintain contact with the tripods of your feet?
Is your weight more on the inside or the outside of your feet?

Notice how the muscles in your upper body respond to this position.
Do you sense muscular effort in your neck and shoulders?
Do you sense effort in your upper or lower back?

Notice how the muscles in your lower body respond to this position.
Do you sense any muscular effort in your upper legs?
Do you sense effort in your lower legs and feet?

Notice your breathing.
Can you breathe comfortably in this position?

Remain in this position and slowly lift your arms, as before.

continued

Notice how lifting your arms in this position affects the muscles in your upper body.

Is there muscular effort in your neck and shoulders?

Do you sense effort in your upper or lower back?

Is it comfortable lifting your arms from this standing position?

Rest.

Again, stand with your feet under your pelvis, distributing your weight equally between both feet. Now begin to slowly side-bend your upper body to the right.

Notice how this position affects your balance and skeletal support.

Do you have a sense of balance in this position?

Do you feel supported by your skeleton?

Are you able to maintain contact with the tripods of your feet?

Is your weight more on the inside or the outside of your feet?

Notice how the muscles in your upper body respond to this position.

Do you sense any muscular effort in your neck and shoulders?

Do you sense effort in your upper or lower back?

Notice how the muscles in your lower body respond to this position.

Do you sense any muscular effort in your upper legs?

Do you sense effort in your lower legs and feet?

Notice your breathing.

Can you breathe comfortably in this position?

Remain in this position and slowly lift your arms, as before.

Notice how lifting your arms in this position affects the muscles in your upper body.

Is there muscular effort in your neck and shoulders?

Do you sense effort in your upper or lower back?

Is it comfortable lifting your arms from this standing position?

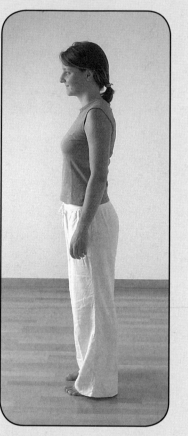

Figure 5.21

Rest.

Standing with your feet under your pelvis and your weight distributed equally between both feet, begin to imagine that you have a string attached to the top, center point of your head. The string is pulling and gently lengthening you, as though you are becoming taller. (5.21)

Now slowly move your upper body as before, a bit forward, backward and side-to-side. Take your time, finding a place where you sense your upper body to be vertically aligned over your pelvis, legs and feet. Once you find your vertical alignment, stand and sense it for a moment.

continued

Tip When you find your vertical alignment, you will feel your weight being distributed throughout your entire body and supported by the tripods of your feet.

Notice how this position affects your balance and skeletal support.
Do you have a have a better sense of balance in this position?
Do you feel supported by your skeleton?
Are you able to maintain contact with the tripods of your feet?

Notice how the muscles in your upper body respond to this position.
Do you sense less muscular effort in your neck and shoulders?
Do you sense less effort in your upper or lower back?

Notice how the muscles in your lower body respond to this position.
Do you sense less muscular effort in your upper legs?
Do you sense less effort in your lower legs and feet?

Notice your breathing.
Can you breathe comfortably in this position?

Remain vertically aligned and lift your arms.

Notice how lifting your arms in this position affects the muscles in your upper body.
Do you sense less muscular effort in your neck and shoulders?
Do you sense less effort in your upper or lower back?
Is it comfortable lifting your arms from this vertical position?

Notice your breathing.
Can you breathe comfortably in this position?

Bring your arms down and continue to stand vertically aligned and enjoy the feeling!

Your body's sense of ease and comfort when standing vertically aligned, is important to remember when adding movements, such as bending, lifting and applying pressure. Though you cannot always stay perfectly aligned, you can maintain a sense of ease and comfort by limiting positions that require extreme effort and cause misalignment.

Self-feedback
How did bending your upper body forward, backward, left and right affect your sense of vertical alignment, balance and support?

_____

What are the advantages of standing vertically aligned?

_____

How can standing vertically aligned improve your body mechanics?

_____

Where's your head?

Balancing your head over your spine is the final step in obtaining a balanced standing posture. Understanding that the head weighs approximately 13 pounds makes it clear as to why it is important to maintain a vertical, balanced head position. Not only is your head relatively heavy, its center of gravity is forward in relation to your spine, causing the muscles at the back of your neck to contract, keeping your head from falling forward.[8] (5.22) It is easy to understand why so many manual therapists express frustration with the stress and fatigue they experience in their necks at the end of the day.

Out of habit, it is common to hold the head in one position. This is not to say that the head does not move out of this position, but in general, there is usually one favorite position in which the head is held, for example, rotated a little bit to the right or left. (5.23) You can find out where you usually hold your head by simply standing and looking into a mirror. While looking, don't change anything about your standing or head position, just notice where, for instance, your nose and eyes are in relation to your center line. As mentioned in Chapter 1, being more aware of your habitual holding patterns is one of the first steps in improving your body mechanics.

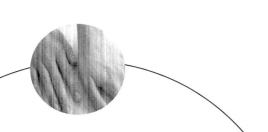

Practice tip 5.5

All of the bones in your body, except your head, have other bones pressing on them. This gives them feedback, telling them where they are in relation to each other and where they are in space. Try to sense where your head is, in relation to the rest of your body, by putting a book (not too heavy) on top of your head. This can help give you a kinesthetic sense of where your head is in space.

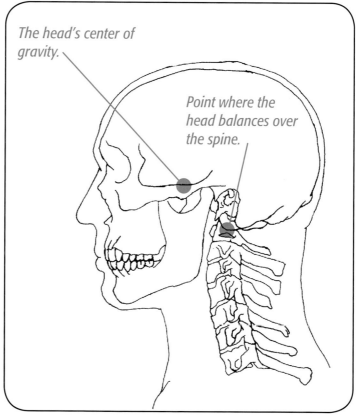

The head's center of gravity.

Point where the head balances over the spine.

Figure 5.22

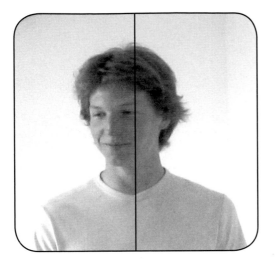

Figure 5.23

Balancing your head over your spine can decrease much of the muscular tension felt in your neck caused from, for example, a forward-head posture. (5.24) When your head is balanced, it is also vertically aligned, giving the rest of your body the perception that your head's weight is very light. (5.25) Standing in a balanced manner by using the tripods of your feet, vertical alignment and proper head balance reduces the stress and strain on your body, allowing it to function more dynamically.

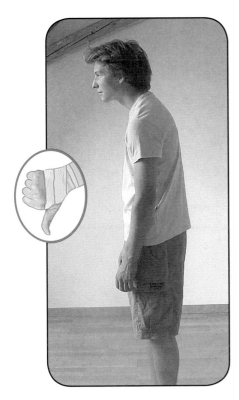

Figure 5.24

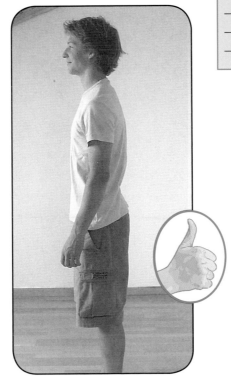

Figure 5.25

Balancing your head over your spine

Stand vertically aligned and bring your attention to your head.

Notice how and where you hold your head.
Do you hold your head with your chin up or down?
Do you hold your head with your chin turned toward your right or left shoulder?
Is your head tilted toward your right or left shoulder?

Imagine that your head is a helium balloon and is floating at the top of your spine. Don't increase your muscular effort to do this. Let your muscles relax and imagine that your head is floating without effort. Begin to slowly move your head up and down, as if you are nodding "yes". Allow your eyes to follow the movement of your head, making very slow and small movements. (5.26)

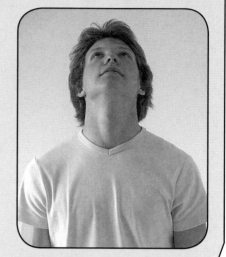

Figure 5.26

Notice what part of your spine you make this movement from.
Do you make this movement from the bottom or the top of your cervical spine?
How high up on your cervical spine can you make this movement?

Tip You may need to make smaller movements in order to feel the movement coming from the top of your spine.

Continue to slowly nod "yes." Make this movement until you find a place somewhere between up and down where you sense your head to be balanced over your shoulders and cervical spine.

Notice the position of your head now.
Does your head feel lighter, as if it is floating about your shoulders?

Rest.

Once again, stand vertically aligned, bringing your attention to your head. Imagine that your head is a helium balloon, sitting at the very top of your spine. Begin to turn your head right and left, as if you are making the movement of "no". Make small and slow movements. (5.27)

Notice what part of your spine you make this movement from.
Do you make this movement from the bottom or the top of your cervical spine?
How high up on your cervical spine can you make this movement?

Continue to slowly turn your head right and left. Make this movement until you find a place somewhere between right and left where you sense your head to be balanced over your shoulders and cervical spine.

continued

Notice the position of your head now.
Is your head balanced on the top of your spine without muscular effort?

Rest.

Stand vertically aligned, bringing your attention to your head. Again, imagine your head as a helium balloon and begin to tilt your head toward your right shoulder and then tilt your head toward your left shoulder. Be sure to make slow and small movements. (5.28)

Continue this movement until you can find a place between your right and left shoulders where your head is balanced over your shoulders and sitting on the top of your spine.

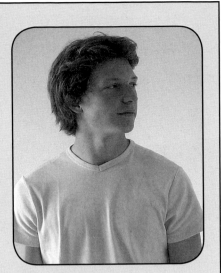

Figure 5.27

Notice the position of your head now.
Is your head balanced on the top of your spine without muscular effort?

Look around and sense the movement of your head.

Notice the quality of movement you now have.
Do you sense a feeling of ease and lightness as you move your head?

Tip Balancing your head over your spine can dramatically reduce the sense of fatigue that you feel in your neck and shoulders at the end of your workday. However, because of the strong holding patterns in the neck, it may take some time to perfect this concept. Try incorporating small parts of this lesson into your body mechanics. Before long you will have a light and free floating head!

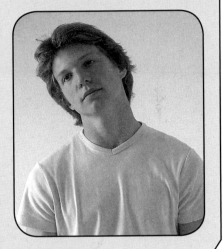

Figure 5.28

Having explored the three *Self-observation* lessons in this chapter, you now know how to use your musculoskeletal system optimally when standing. The concepts learned give you the means to reduce muscular tension, increase comfort and work in a balanced standing posture.

Self-feedback
Regarding the last three Self-observation lessons:
How have they influenced your standing posture?

_____
_____

What concepts did you find most beneficial to you?

_____
_____
_____

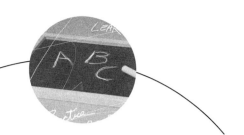

Client education tip 5.4

If a client is experiencing discomfort in the neck, notice if she or he holds the head out in front of the spine and shoulders. As you know, this creates a lot of work for the muscles of the neck, causing discomfort. Help your client find a more balanced position over the spine by leading him or her through Self-observation 5.3. If necessary, take a few sessions to complete the lesson - a little goes a long way!

Summary

In this chapter, you have explored how to stand supported by your musculoskeletal system. You have learned how to use the tripods of your feet, vertically balance your upper body over your lower body and balance your head over your spine. Here's a review of the concepts learned in the chapter:

Standing can be defined as a basic functional posture from which all other body mechanics can be performed, for example, lifting, bending, pushing, pulling and applying pressure. With a **balanced standing** posture, stability and dynamic movements allow you to effectively execute the specific functions of manual therapy.

Learning to find a balanced standing posture begins with utilizing the **"tripods" of your feet**. When properly utilized, your foot's tripod can support, distribute and absorb your body's weight. When using a **stance**, make sure both feet are pointed toward your direction of movement to decrease the risk of strain to your back, knees and ankles. Your stance should transmit the weight of your body evenly down to your feet, allowing you to engage the tripods of your feet, increasing the overall stability of your stance. Keep your body **vertically aligned** over your pelvis, legs and feet. When vertical, the force of gravity is distributed throughout your entire body, allowing all the joints in your body to effortlessly support you. **Balancing your head** over your spine is the final detail. A balanced head posture decreases much of the muscular tension felt in your neck caused from, for example, a forward-head posture. When your head is balanced, it is also vertically aligned, giving the rest of your body the perception that your head's weight is very light.

Now that you've read this chapter...

How aware are you now of your standing habits?

- almost always
- sometimes
- not very often
- other_____

What parts of your body are you most aware of now when standing?

- neck and shoulders
- arms and hands
- lower back and feet
- other_____

What parts of your body are you still not aware of?

- neck and shoulders
- arms and hands
- lower back and feet
- other_____

Describe 5 concepts that make your standing more dynamic.

1. _____
2. _____
3. _____
4. _____
5. _____

Describe an aspect of standing that feels easy and comfortable.

(e.g., standing on the "tripods" of your feet.)

_____

_____

Describe an aspect of standing that you don't feel comfortable with yet.

_____

_____

Now how comfortable are you standing?

- completely
- mostly
- a little
- not very

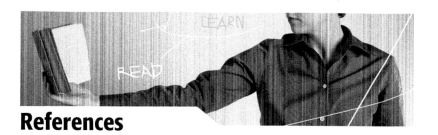

References

1. Chester, John. *Personal Communication.* Feldenkrais Professional Training Program. Seattle, WA, 1999.

2. Todd, Mabel E. *The Thinking Body.* Brooklyn: Dance Horizons/Princeton Book Co., 1979.

3. Muscolino, Joseph E. *Electronic Communication.* June 2003.

4. Biel, Andrew. *Trail Guide to the Body, 2nd Edition.* Boulder: Books of Discovery, 2001.

5. Haller, Jeff. *Feldenkrais Professional Training Program.* Maui, Hawaii, 1994.

6. Todd, Mabel E. *The Thinking Body.* Brooklyn: Dance Horizons/Princeton Book Co., 1979.

7. Muscolino, Joseph E. *Electronic Communication.* June 2003.

8. Brennan, Richard. *The Alexander Technique Workbook.* Shaftesbury: Element Books Limited,1992.

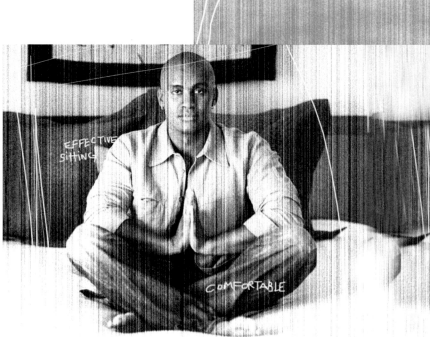

6 Sitting

Introduction

As with standing, sitting is also a basic functional posture. Unlike standing, however, sitting requires you to remain on a chair while executing other functions, such as lifting, pushing and pulling. Because our bodies are structured for a bi-pedal life, sitting comfortably presents a challenge—but don't worry. Though the pelvis is oddly shaped and primarily functional for walking, it provides an efficient sitting platform. With help from the legs and feet, it is possible to sit comfortably for long periods of time.

In this chapter, you will learn about the important roles the pelvis, legs and feet play in proper sitting. We will continue our discussion of vertical alignment and head balance with regard to sitting. Knee height and leg width will also be discussed. Ultimately, you will learn to sit in a way that will support and give you the freedom to perform your manual therapy dynamically and effectively.

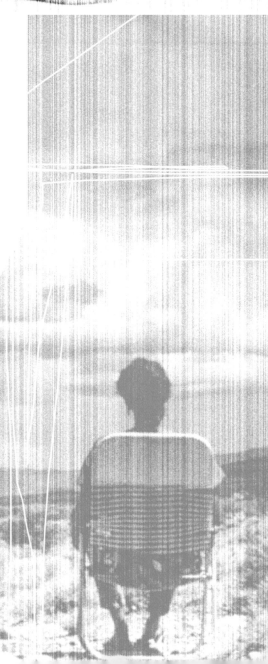

Before you read this chapter…

How often do you sit on a daily basis?
- *almost always*
- *sometimes*
- *not very often*
- *other_____*

What parts of your body are you most aware of when sitting?
- *head and neck*
- *shoulders and upper back*
- *pelvis and legs*
- *other_____*

What parts of your body are you least aware of when sitting?
- *head and neck*
- *shoulders and upper back*
- *pelvis and legs*
- *other_____*

Describe 5 sitting habits that you are aware of on a daily basis.
(e.g., do you usually sit with your legs crossed?)
1. _____
2. _____
3. _____
4. _____
5. _____

Describe an everyday activity involving sitting that you do with ease and comfort.
_____
_____

Describe an everyday activity involving sitting that you do with difficulty or discomfort.
_____
_____

How comfortable are you sitting on an everyday basis?
- *always*
- *mostly*
- *sometimes*
- *very seldom*

Balanced sitting

A poor sitting posture is one of three factors commonly seen in people with low back pain.[1] Frequent flexion (bending forward at the waist) and the inability to fully extend (bend backwards) are the other two, both of which we will address later in this book. Given that sitting, like standing, is a basic functional posture of manual therapy, it is crucial to learn how to sit with a balanced, thus, healthy posture.

Depending on the type of manual therapy, sitting can be the main functional posture or used intermittently. For example, a therapist working primarily with the head and neck will sit during most of her sessions. On the other hand, a therapist giving a full-body relaxation massage will sit only for a short time. However, whether for a short or long period of time, sitting, for a manual therapist, is not as simple as it may seem. You are usually performing other movements when sitting, e.g., reaching, bending, pushing and pulling. Being in constant movement requires you to have a sitting posture that not only protects your low back, but also allows you to be mobile. Sitting in a balanced manner allows your musculoskeletal system to support you, decreasing pressure on the low back, specifically the intervertebral discs. In addition, it gives you the ability to perform the techniques of your therapy effectively.

Sitting with a balanced posture means your pelvis, legs and feet support you, your upper body is vertically aligned and your head is balanced over your spine. (6.1) With these attributes, although you are "fixed" to a chair, your spine, especially your low back, is put under less strain than when, for example, sitting in a "slouched" posture. (6.2) Balanced sitting allows the natural curvature of your spine and your lower body to support you, decreasing strain and increasing your effectiveness.

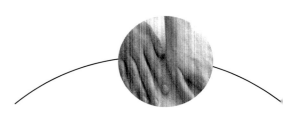

Practice tip 6.1

The next time you are working in a seated position, notice where you tend to place your legs and feet. Notice if your legs are crossed, out in front of you or tucked up underneath your chair. Do you place one foot on the floor and the other on your chair? Explore placing both feet on the ground for support and becoming more aware of your "tripods" (see Standing, Ch. 5, pg.113) Using both feet on the ground will decrease the effort in your legs and help make sitting more comfortable.

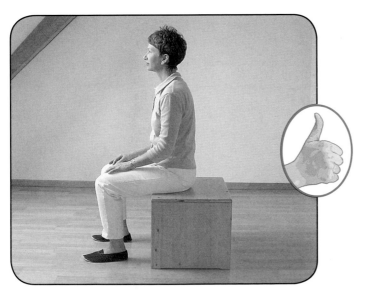

Figure 6.1

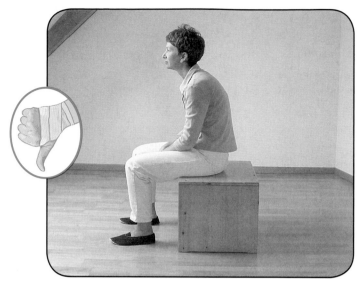

Figure 6.2

The pelvis, leg and foot connection

Using the pelvis, legs and feet for support is the first step toward a balanced sitting posture. Let's take a look at the pelvis. The structure of your pelvis can be compared to a bowl. (6.3) At its base are the ischial tuberosities, commonly called the "sit-bones", on which your skeleton can rest when sitting. You are probably more aware of your pelvis than, for instance, your legs or feet when sitting. That's because most of your body's weight is put on your pelvis. It is important to note that, when sitting in a balanced manner, the ischial tuberosities are the proper points of contact, not the coccyx. Because most people put weight on the coccyx when sitting, it is easy to think of it as a "sit-bone". But, in reality, the coccyx is considered part of the spine and no weight should be placed upon it. Becoming aware of your ischial tuberosities and supporting your weight with them takes the pressure off your low back. However, your legs, specifically the upper posterior thighs, also play an important role in supporting your body.

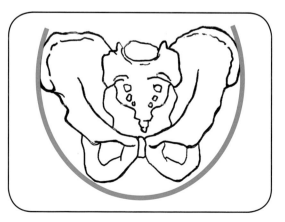

Figure 6.3

Your legs share your body's weight and stabilize it from tipping over. Without your legs, it would be very difficult for your pelvis to stabilize you while sitting. Can you imagine sitting without the support of your legs? When the legs are used efficiently, weight is distributed over the pelvis and posterior thighs, taking stress off the spine. This relieves much of the strain and fatigue felt in the low back. And last, but not least, your feet do the rest. Because of their position on the floor, they stabilize and counterbalance your body's weight. The connection of your feet to your legs makes it possible for you to sit with a solid connection to your chair and floor.

Ultimately, the connection between your chair, pelvis, legs, feet and floor allows you to sit with a balanced posture, increasing your stability and effectiveness. (6.4)

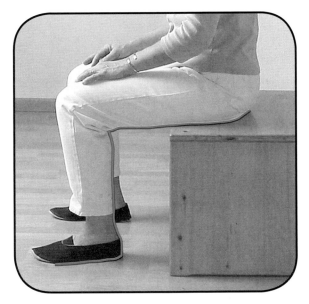

Figure 6.4

The following *Self-observation* lesson will help you experience this concept.

Something to think about...

Why and how often do you sit during a session?

_____
_____

Is your back, especially low back, comfortable when sitting? Explain.

_____
_____

How aware are you of your ischial tuberosities, legs and feet when sitting?

_____
_____

What are some things you can do to help remind yourself to sit in a balanced manner?

_____
_____
_____

Making the pelvis, leg and foot connection

Sit on a flat, firm surface. Place your legs approximately hip-width apart, with your ankles underneath your knees. Sit with your spine in a neutral position, not flexed forward or extended backward. Now, begin to tilt your pelvis a little bit forward and backward.

Tip Your ischial tuberosities are shaped like the base of a rocking chair and can easily rock or tilt your pelvis forward and backward. (6.5)
Can you feel your ischial tuberosities moving on the surface of your chair or stool?

Tip Place your hand underneath your pelvis while continuing to move. This will help you feel the structure of the tuberosities.

Once you have a clear tactile sense, take your hand away and continue to roll your pelvis back and forth until you have a clear idea of what it feels like to sit on your ischial tuberosities.

Rest.

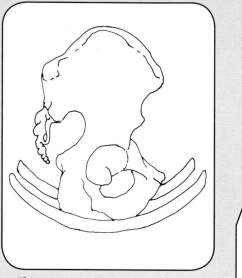

Figure 6.5

Sit again with your spine in a neutral position, on your ischial tuberosities. Place your legs approximately hip-width apart, with your ankles underneath your knees. Slowly begin to round your upper body, bringing your head, neck, shoulders and back into flexion. (6.6)

Notice how your flexed position influences the position of the ischial tuberosities.
*How does flexing your upper body change the contact between the ischial tuberosities and your sitting surface? Is the contact as clear as it was when sitting in a neutral position?
Do you feel supported by your ischial tuberosities now?*

Notice how your body responds to this position.
*How does your low back respond to this position?
What part of your pelvis is your weight resting on?
Is your weight resting on the coccyx and sacrum?*

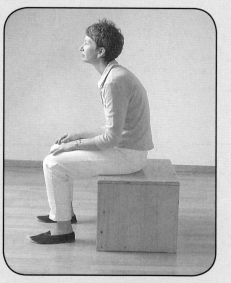

Figure 6.6

continued

How much weight is on your thighs?
How much weight is on your feet?
Is this sitting position one that you use often?

Rest.

Sit as before. Slowly begin to hyperextend your upper body. (6.7)

Notice how your extended position influences the position of the ischial tuberosities.
How does flexing your upper body change the contact between the ischial tuberosities and your sitting surface?
Is the contact as clear as it was when sitting in a neutral position?
Do you feel supported by your ischial tuberosities now?

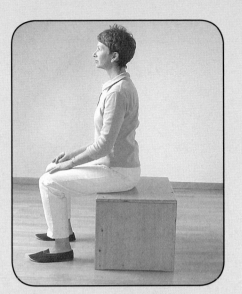

Figure 6.7

Notice how your body responds to this position.
How does your low back respond to this position?
What part of your pelvis is your weight resting on?
How much weight is on your thighs?
How much weight is on your feet?
Is this position one that you use often?

Rest.

Once again, sit with your spine in a neutral position, on your ischial tuberosities. Place your legs hip-width apart, with your ankles underneath your knees. (6.8)

Notice how sitting in a neutral position allows fuller contact between your ischial tuberosities and your sitting surface.
Why does this position allow for more contact to the sitting surface?

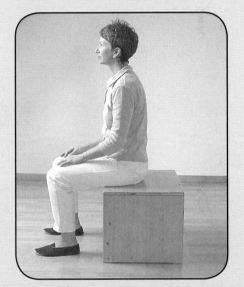

Figure 6.8

Is the contact between your sitting surface and ischial tuberosities clearer in this sitting position than in a flexed or hyperextended position?
Do you feel fully supported by your ischial tuberosities now?

Notice how this neutral sitting position changes how your body feels.
How does your low back respond to this position?
What part of your pelvis is your weight resting on?
How much weight is on your upper legs?
How much weight is on your feet?
Is this neutral position one that you use on a regular basis?

continued

Rest.

Once again, sit as before. Bring your attention to your upper legs and their contact to the chair. Let your legs share the weight of your body with your ischial tuberosities.

Notice how your legs support your body's weight.
Do you sense how your thighs and ischial tuberosities support you?
How much weight is on your legs?
Is it comfortable to rest your weight on your pelvis and legs?

Notice how your back responds to this position.
Is your lower back able to relax, allowing your pelvis and legs to support you?
Do you feel less effort in your mid and upper back?

Rest.

Sit as before. Bring your attention to your feet and their contact to the floor. Let your feet stabilize your body and share the remaining weight.

Tip Placing your ankles underneath your knees increases your skeletal support and decreases the muscular effort in your legs *(see Partner practice 1.1).*

Notice how your feet act to stabilize and support your body's weight.
Do you sense how your feet stabilize your body?
How much weight is on your feet?

Notice how your back responds to this position.
Is your lower back able to relax, allowing your pelvis, thighs and feet to support you?
Do you feel less effort in your mid and upper back?

Rest.

Once again, sit as before. Bring your attention to the skeletal support you have now created. (6.9)

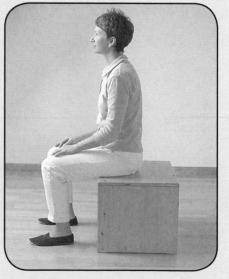

Figure 6.9

continued

Notice how your body responds to using your pelvis, legs and feet for support.

Do you sense less muscular effort in your back?

Does this feel like a position that you can sit in for a long period of time?

Does it feel like a position that you will need to get used to using?

Does it feel like a sitting position that you have used in the past?

Using your pelvis, legs and feet to create a base of support is the most effective way to sit and work. It reduces your muscular effort and allows your body to move in a more dynamic way. However, this may be a very new way for you to sit and at first may feel strange - if not tiring. Take your time to become comfortable with this new way of sitting. If you begin to feel tired or strained, relax into a more familiar sitting position, coming back to the new way when ready.

Self-feedback

How does sitting with your pelvis, legs and feet in this manner affect your overall sitting comfort?

_____

_____

How does this new sitting position compare to other sitting postures you have used?

_____

_____

Will you use this new sitting position? Explain.

_____

_____

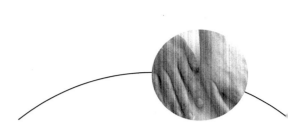

Practice tip 6.2

When you feel uncomfortable sitting during a session, take a few minutes and sense where your spine is in relation to your pelvis. Notice if it is flexed (slouched) forward or extended backward. If so, bring yourself back into a neutral position, finding a place where your spine feels comfortable, and your pelvis, legs and feet support you. Finding your skeletal support will quickly relieve muscular strain and effort.

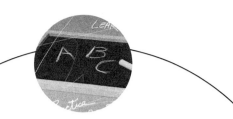

Sitting vertically aligned

Sitting with a vertically aligned posture is the next step toward achieving balance. When vertically aligned, the natural curvature of your spine is in a neutral position, not too flexed or extended, and your upper body's relationship with your pelvis is vertical, not too forward or backward. (6.10)

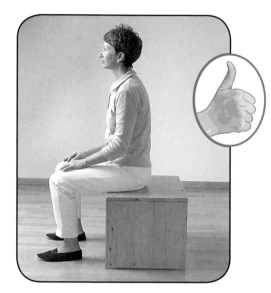

Figure 6.10

As you have experienced with standing, vertical alignment allows your spine to maintain its natural curves and to distribute effort proportionally, so no part overworks while others are stressed. When sitting with your weight distributed over your pelvis, legs and feet, your spine can easily remain in neutral instead of buckling forward or arching backward in the attempt to support weight and maintain stability. Thus, with your spine in a neutral, vertical position, it is easier to establish a vertical relationship between your upper body and pelvis.[2]

When sitting, your center of gravity is lowered and your base of support is larger than when standing. Sitting on a large base of support instead of standing on a small one gives you more stability but, because of the wider base, it is much easier to collapse into a "slouched" or forward posture. (6.11) Slouching forward may feel comfortable at first, but after a few moments your body becomes fatigued and thus restless in its attempt to find a more comfortable position. The next time you are sitting with a group of people, observe all of the different sitting postures. Find someone who seems comfortable and has no problem sitting in the same position for a long period of time. Notice where they place their feet and if they are vertically aligned.

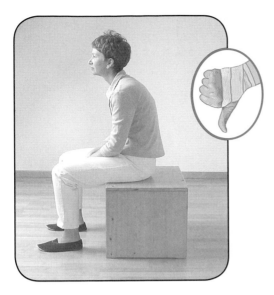

Figure 6.11

The bottom line is, the more comfortable you are sitting, the more effective your therapy will be. Whether or not you feel a sense of stability, you will more than likely feel a sense of comfort. Your sensory cues will help you recognize your comfort zone – and chances are it will involve vertical alignment.

The following *Self-observation* lesson helps to highlight the advantages of sitting vertically aligned.

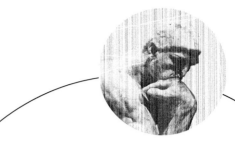

Consider this

Muscle tension of the posterior neck is increased by 50 percent when sitting in a forward flexed position.[3]

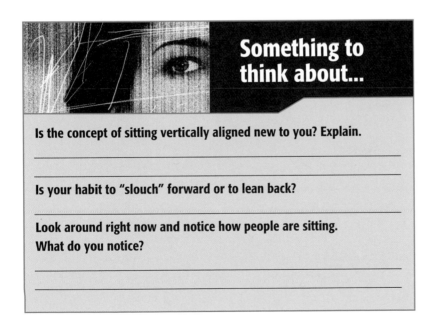

Something to think about...

Is the concept of sitting vertically aligned new to you? Explain.

_____

_____

Is your habit to "slouch" forward or to lean back?

_____

Look around right now and notice how people are sitting. What do you notice?

_____

_____

Sitting with vertical alignment

Sit on a flat, firm surface and place your feet on the floor so that your ankles are under your knees. Your knees should be approximately at hip height and hip width apart. Begin to roll or tilt your pelvis back and let your back, shoulders and head flex forward. (6.12)

Tip This movement is very similar to "slumping" down in a chair. In this position your upper body is collapsing so that your spine has little chance to support you.

Notice how your body responds to this position.
Do you sense that your upper body and pelvis are not vertically aligned in this position?
Do you sense that your thoracic curve has increased and lumbar curve decreased?

Notice how the muscles in your back respond to this flexed position.
Do you feel muscular tension in your lower back?
Do you feel tension in your mid and upper back?

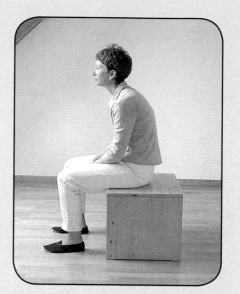

Figure 6.12

Notice your breathing.
Can you breathe comfortably in this position?

Tip In this position, movement of your diaphragm is restricted, making it hard for you to breathe normally.

Remain in this position and slowly raise your arms in front of you. (6.13)

Notice how your body responds to this movement.
Do you feel a sense of effort?
Do you sense effort in your shoulders?
Do you sense effort in your back?
Do you sense effort in your neck?
Does this feel like a position that you work in?

Rest.

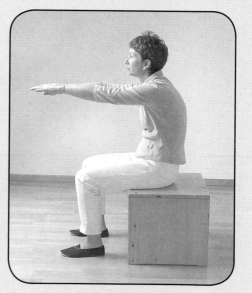

Figure 6.13

continued

Sit again, as before. Begin to roll or tilt your pelvis forward. Let your back, shoulders and head extend backward. (6.14)

Tip This movement should feel as if you are arching your back.

Notice how your body responds to this position.
Do you sense that your upper body and pelvis are not vertically aligned in this position?
Can you sense that your thoracic curve has decreased and lumbar curve increased?

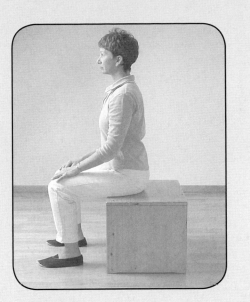

Figure 6.14

Notice how the muscles in your back respond to this arched position.
Do you feel muscular tension in your lower back?
Do you feel tension in your mid and upper back?
Are your shoulders forced backward?

Notice your breathing.
Can you breathe comfortably in this position?

Remain in this position and raise your arms, as before. (6.15)

Notice how your body responds to this movement.
Do you feel a sense of effort?
Do you sense effort in your shoulders?
Do you sense effort in your back?
Do you sense effort in your neck?
Is this a familiar working position?

Rest.

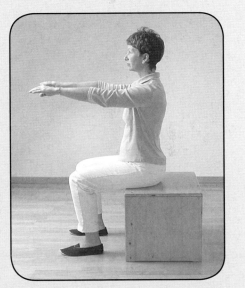

Figure 6.15

continued

Sit again, as before. Begin to roll or tilt your pelvis to a place where you sense it resting on its base and where your weight is supported by your pelvis, legs and feet. Allow your back, shoulders and head to move with the tilting movement of your pelvis so that you eventually find a place where your upper body feels vertically aligned with your pelvis. (6.16)

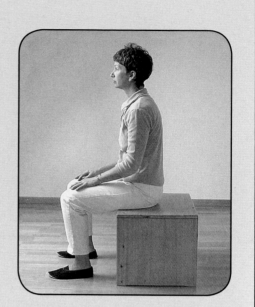

Figure 6.16

Tip This will be a neutral position, somewhere between the backward and forward movements previously made.

Notice the relation between your upper body and pelvis.
Do you sense that your upper body and pelvis are vertically aligned in this position?
Do you sense that your thoracic and lumbar spine are in a neutral position?

Notice how the muscles in your back respond to this vertical alignment.
Do you sense less muscular tension in your lower back?
Do you sense less tension in your mid and upper back?
Are your shoulders more comfortable?

Notice your breathing.
Can you breathe more comfortably in this position?

Remain in this position and raise your arms, as before. (6.17)

Notice how your body responds to this movement.
Do you feel a sense of ease while raising your arms?
Do you sense more ease in your shoulders?
Do you sense more ease in your back?
Do you sense more ease in your neck?
Is this a familiar working position?

Lower your arms and continue to sit for a few minutes. Enjoy the feeling of sitting in a vertically aligned and comfortable manner.

Becoming more aware of the relationship between your pelvis and upper body and maintaining their alignment, gives you a sense of stability and mobility. The underlying sense of comfort will increase the effectiveness and success of your treatments.

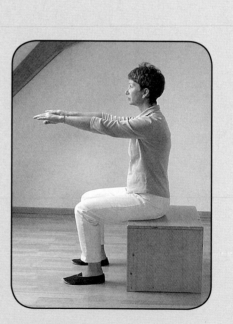

Figure 6.17

continued

Self-observation 6.2, continued

Self-feedback

What differences did you notice when lifting your arms with a flexed, an extended and a vertically aligned posture?

_____

_____

What differences did you notice with regard to the comfort of your back?

_____

_____

What differences did you notice in your breathing?

_____

_____

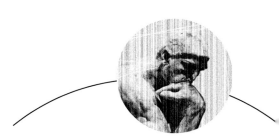

Consider this

"The posture of an anteriorly held head requires all of the extensor musculature in the posterior neck to chronically tighten isometrically to hold the head from falling forward down to the chest due to the pull of gravity. For this reason, this type of posture creates tight neck musculature. If left untreated, these tight posterior neck muscles often lead to tension headaches and, in time may even lead to TMJ dysfunction." [4]

Dr. Joseph E. Muscolino

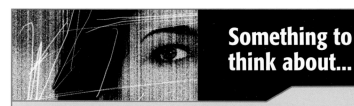

Something to think about...

When working in a sitting position, how do you habitually hold your head?

_____

_____

Do you sense the weight of your head when sitting? Explain.

_____

How comfortable are your neck and shoulders when working?

_____

_____

Are your neck and shoulders places that typically become stiff after a day's work?

_____

_____

Where's your head? - the sequel...

A balanced head posture is the next step toward achieving a fully balanced sitting posture.

As you have learned, the head is relatively heavy and its center of gravity is anterior in relation to your spine. When sitting, your head's weight and position is a bit easier to negotiate because of the wide base of support given by the pelvis and legs. However, when sitting, it is just as important to balance your head properly over your spine to have a sense of comfort and ease while working. (6.18) With proper head balance, the muscles of the neck, especially the extensor musculature in the posterior neck, work less. Less muscular work means more comfort for you.

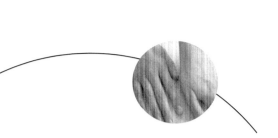

Practice tip 6.3

The next time you find yourself sitting in a forward, flexed position, try looking up toward the ceiling. Notice how much range of motion you have in your neck as you look up. You will probably find that your neck is limited in its movement when sitting in a forward, flexed posture. After exploring this, sit vertically aligned with your head balanced over your spine and look up again. You will most likely sense that you have much more range of motion and perhaps you will even see more of the ceiling!

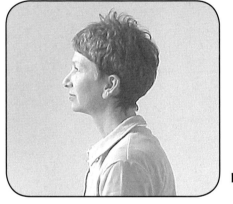

Figure 6.18

Upper back and neck pain and tension are common complaints among manual therapists who sit while working. Naturally, a goal of most manual therapists is to reduce the amount of tension felt. This goal is not difficult to achieve, but the first step is finding out how you habitually hold your head while sitting:

Take a moment now and sit the way you normally would when working. For example, sit at the end of your table as if to work with a client's head, neck or feet. Notice if your tendency is to sit with your head held out in front of yourself or with it held back. Is your habit to hold your head to one side? Do you hold your head in a side-bent position and/or rotated?

Discovering what your habitual holding pattern is will help you understand why you perhaps experience neck fatigue during or after your sessions. This awareness will also assist you in finding a more neutral, balanced position with which you can experience comfort and ease.

The previous two *Self-observation* lessons taught you how to feel the support of your pelvis, legs and feet, and to experience vertical alignment. The following *Self-observation* lesson will give you the opportunity to explore a balanced head posture.

Finding your head's balance.

Sit in a neutral position, with your weight on your ischial tuberosities, legs and feet, and vertically aligned. Your knees should be approximately at hip height and hip width apart.

Notice where your head is.
Do you sense where your head is in relation to your shoulders?
Do you sense where it is in relation to your upper back?
Do you sense where it is in relation to your pelvis?

Move your head out in front of your shoulders, so that your chin comes away from your throat. (6.19)

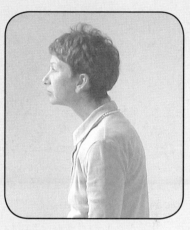

Figure 6.19

Tip If needed, put your hand on top of your head and see if it helps you sense where your head is in relation to the rest of your body.

Notice the weight of your head in this forward position.
Does it feel heavy?
How does the weight and position of your head affect your neck?
How does the weight and position of your head affect your upper back?
How does the weight and position of your head affect your shoulders?
How does the weight and position of your head influence your breathing?

Leave your head in front of your shoulders and lift your arms up. (6.20)

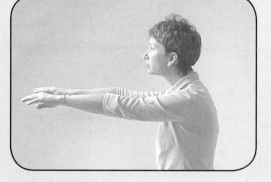

Notice how your body responds to lifting your arms with a forward head position.
Is it easy or difficult to lift your arms?
How does lifting your arms with your head forward affect the muscles in your neck?
How does lifting your arms with your head forward affect the muscles in your upper back?
How does lifting your arms affect the muscles in your shoulders?

Figure 6.20

continued

Notice your breathing.
How does lifting your arms with your head in this position affect your breathing?
Is it easy or difficult to breathe?

With your head forward and your arms raised, move your head slowly and look around the room.

Notice how it feels to move your head in this position.
Is it easy or difficult to move your head?

Rest.

Sit once again, as before. Move your head back, so that
your chin comes closer to your throat. (6.21)

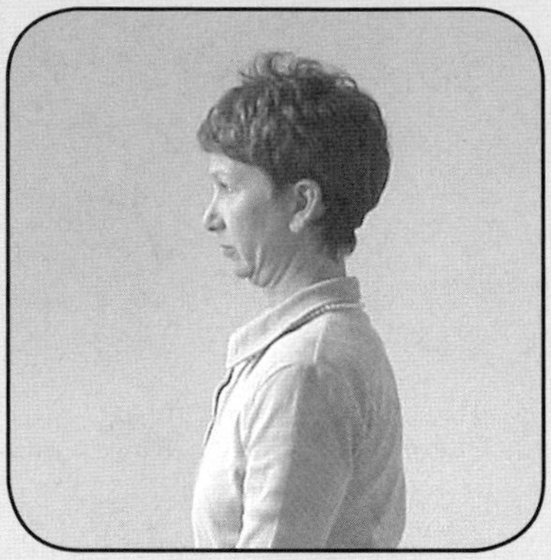

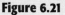

Figure 6.21

Notice the weight of your head in this position.
Does it feel heavy?
How does your head's weight and position now affect your neck?
How does your head's weight and position affect your upper back?
How does your head's weight and position affect your shoulders?
How does your head's weight and position influence your breathing?

Leave your head in this position and lift your arms up. (6.22)

Notice how lifting your arms with a posterior head position affects your body.
Is it easy or difficult to lift your arms?
How does lifting your arms from this position affect the muscles in your neck?
How does lifting your arms from this position affect the muscles in your upper back?
How does lifting your arms affect the muscles in your shoulders?

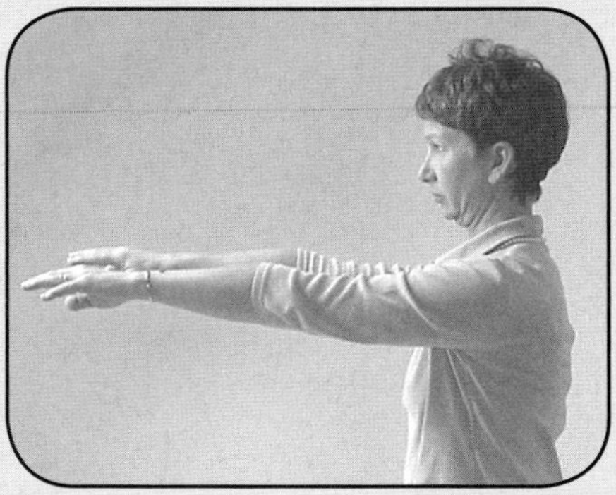

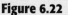

Figure 6.22

Notice your breathing.
How does lifting your arms from this position affect your breathing?
Is it easy or difficult to breathe?

With your arms raised and your head back, move your head slowly and look around the room.

Notice how it feels to move your head.
Is it easy or difficult to move your head from this position?

Rest.

continued

Sit again as before. Move your head until you find a place where your head feels balanced over your spine. (6.23)

Tip This place will be somewhere between the anterior and posterior positions you have just explored. Don't feel frustrated if at first it is difficult for you to find a balanced place for your head. Just take your time and make very small movements.

Notice the weight of your head in this balanced position.
Does it feel lighter?
Do you have a sense of ease in your neck?
Do you have a sense of less effort in your upper back?
How does the lightness of your head and its position affect your shoulders?
Does the balanced position of your head increase your ability to breathe?

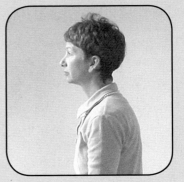

Figure 6.23

Now leave your head in this balanced position and lift your arms. (6.24)

Notice how your body responds to lifting your arms with a balanced head position.
Is it easier to lift your arms?
How does lifting your arms now affect the muscles in your neck?
How does lifting your arms affect the muscles in your upper back?
How does lifting your arms affect the muscles in your shoulders?

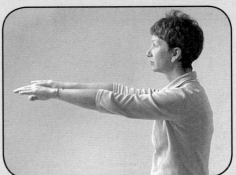

Figure 6.24

Notice your breathing.
How does lifting your arms with a balanced head position affect your breathing?
Is it easier to breathe now?

With your arms raised, move your head slowly and look around the room.

Tip If your head is balanced, you will sense very little muscular tension in your neck while moving your head.

Notice how it feels to move your head.
Is it easy or difficult to move your head from this position?

continued

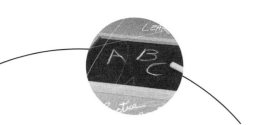

Client education tip 6.2

If a client is experiencing discomfort in their upper back and neck when sitting, notice the position of his or her head. Chances are it is not balanced over the spine, creating work for the muscles of the upper back and neck. Help your client find a more balanced position by leading him or her through Self-observation 6.3. Point out that when the head's heavy weight is over the spine, it becomes seemingly weightless.

Lower your arms and continue to sit with your head balanced over your spine. Enjoy the feeling of lightness you have in your head and its effect on your neck, back, shoulders and breathing.

Using the support of your pelvis, legs and feet, vertical alignment and head balance when sitting dramatically increases your comfort and effectiveness. Your musculoskeletal system fully supports you, increasing your stability and mobility.

Self-feedback
How did the different head positions explored in this lesson affect the overall comfort of your neck, back and shoulder?

_____

_____

Has the awareness of your head's weight and its effect on your body increased? Explain.

_____

_____

How and why did the different head positions explored affect your breathing?

_____

_____

Knee height and leg width

Because of its connection to your legs, the position of your pelvis in sitting is greatly determined by the height of your knees and the width your legs. Thus finding the optimal knee height and leg width are the final keys to a balanced sitting posture.

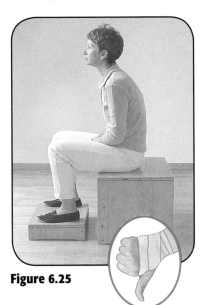

Figure 6.25

When sitting, it is important that your knees are the same height as your hips. When your knees are higher than your hips, your pelvis is forced back and the vertical alignment of your pelvis and upper body is compromised. With the knees higher, you are forced into a "slouched" position. (6.25) When your knees are lower than your hips, your pelvis automatically rolls forward and again, your vertical alignment is compromised. A forced arching of the back is experienced when the knees are lower than the pelvis. (6.26) Keep your knees approximately at the height of your hips to increase the comfort and effectiveness of your sitting. In this position, your pelvis is able to maintain a neutral position and your back is allowed to stay in vertical alignment, not forced forward or back. (6.27)

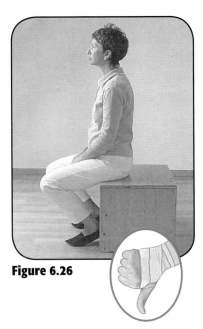

Figure 6.26

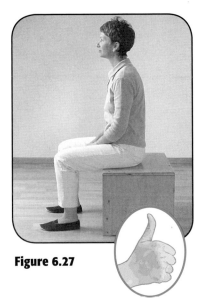

Figure 6.27

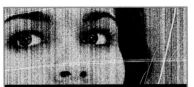

Something to think about...

When working in a sitting position:
In general, how high or low are your knees?

_____
_____
_____

Can your feet comfortably touch the floor?

_____
_____
_____

In general, how wide apart are your legs?

_____
_____
_____

Does the structure of your table influence how wide apart you hold your legs? Explain.

_____
_____
_____
_____
_____
_____

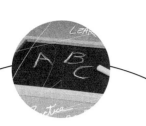

Client education tip 6.3

Women often sit with their legs close together, having been told that sitting with the legs apart is not "ladylike". This sitting posture can cause undue tension in the low back, not allowing the ischial tuberosities to contact the sitting surface adequately. If you have a client with this posture who is experiencing back pain, gently explain this concept to her. Encourage her to explore the difference between her present leg position and a slightly wider one. Your client may not be willing to change her posture, but at least she will be aware of another choice.

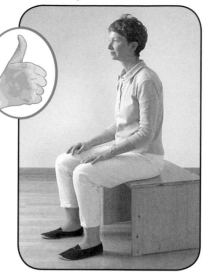

Figure 6.28

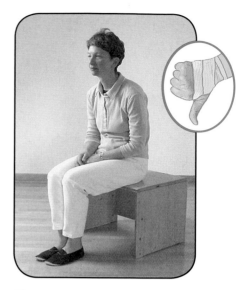

Figure 6.29

The width of your legs also influences the position of your pelvis, which greatly affects your muscular tension, stability and vertical alignment. Your legs' width should be approximately that of your hips. (6.28) Holding your legs too close together usually causes the pelvis to tilt back, creating undue muscular tension in the muscles of the leg. (6.29) Spreading your legs too wide apart usually causes the pelvis to roll forward and creates tension in the abductor muscles of the leg, as well as the gluteals and hip rotators. (6.30) If you find that you need to work with your legs spread wider than your hip's width, take care not to arch your low back and maintain contact between your sitting surface and ischial tuberosities.

The following *Self-observation* lesson will help illuminate the benefits of sitting with proper knee height and leg width.

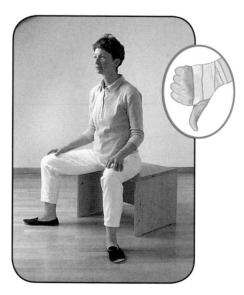

Figure 6.30

Finding the best knee height and leg width.

Sit on a flat, firm surface with your legs close together and your feet on something that brings your knees higher than your hips. (6.31)

Notice how this position affects the quality of your sitting.
Is your pelvis rolled forward or backward?
Can you feel the muscles of your legs working hard to stay together?
Does this sitting position create a stable base of support?
Is this a position that you usually work in?

Rest.

Now sit with your knees lower than your hips and your legs wide apart. (6.32)

Notice how this position affects the quality of your sitting.
Is your pelvis rolled forward or backward?
Do you feel the muscles of your legs working hard to stay apart?
Do you feel stress in your gluteals and hip rotators?
Does this sitting position create a stable base of support?
Can you maintain contact with your ischial tuberosities?
Is this a position that you usually work in?

Rest.

Now sit with your knees approximately hip height and legs hip width apart. (6.33)

Notice how this position affects the quality of your sitting.
Is your pelvis rolled forward, backward or is it in a neutral position?
Do you sense the muscles of your legs working less?
Do you sense the gluteals and hip rotators working less?
Does this sitting position create a stable base of support?

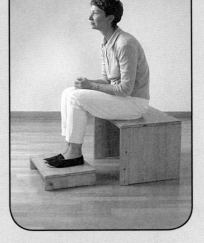

Figure 6.31

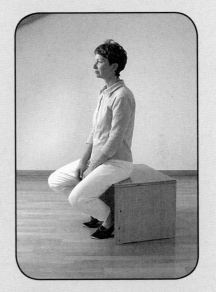

Figure 6.32

continued

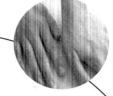

Practice tip 6.4

If you have cause to straddle your table while working, keep your back in a neutral position and maintain contact between your table and ischial tuberosities. Sitting with the legs too wide creates a tendency to hyperextend the spine, and if held for long periods of time, can cause general discomfort in your body. With your back and pelvis in neutral, you decrease stress and allow for a more comfortable posture.

Can you maintain contact with your ischial tuberosities? Is this a position that you usually work in?

Continue sitting in this position for a few minutes, feeling the advantages of sitting with your knees hip-height and legs hip-width apart.

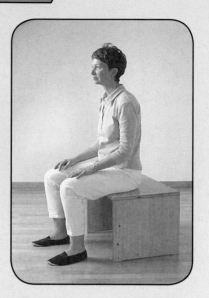

Figure 6.33

Having experienced the four Self-observation lessons in this chapter, you now know how to use your musculoskeletal system optimally when sitting. The concepts learned give you the means to reduce muscular tension, increase comfort and work in a balanced sitting posture.

Self-feedback

Regarding the last four Self-observation lessons:
How have they influenced your sitting posture?

_____

_____

What concepts did you find most beneficial to you?

_____

_____

Now that you've read this chapter…

When working, how aware are you of your sitting habits?
- almost always
- sometimes
- not very often
- other_____

When sitting, what parts of your body are you now most aware of?
- neck and shoulders
- arms and hands
- pelvis and legs
- other_____

When sitting, what parts of your body are you still not aware of?
- neck and shoulders
- arms and hands
- pelvis and legs
- other_____

Describe 5 concepts that make your sitting more balanced.
1. _____
2. _____
3. _____
4. _____
5. _____

Describe an aspect of sitting that feels easy and comfortable.
_____
_____

Describe an aspect of sitting that you don't feel comfortable with yet.
_____
_____

Now how comfortable are you sitting?
- completely
- mostly
- a little
- not at all

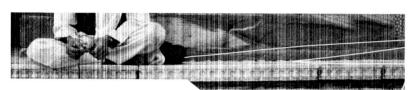

Summary

In this chapter, you have learned about the important roles the pelvis, legs and feet play in proper sitting, and we have continued our discussion of vertical alignment and head balance with regard to sitting. Knee height and leg width were also discussed. Ultimately, you learned how to sit in a balanced sitting manner, giving you the freedom to perform your manual therapy dynamically and effectively. Here is a review of the concepts covered in this chapter:

Balanced sitting means your pelvis, legs and feet support you, your upper body is vertically aligned, your head is balanced over your spine, and knees and legs are at hip height and hip width apart.

Using your **pelvis, legs and feet** to create a base of support is the most effective way to sit and work. It reduces your muscular effort and allows your body to move in a more dynamic way.

Becoming more aware of the relationship between your pelvis and upper body and maintaining their **vertical alignment**, gives you a sense of stability and mobility. The underlying sense of comfort will increase the effectiveness and the success of your treatments.

The head's appreciable weight is seemingly light when balanced over the spine. Thus, proper **head balance** increases a sense of comfort when sitting and reduces muscular tension.

Because of its connection to your legs, the position of your pelvis in sitting is greatly determined by **your knee height and leg width**. Sitting with your knees at hip height and with your legs hip width apart, will increase your overall sense of balance and comfort.

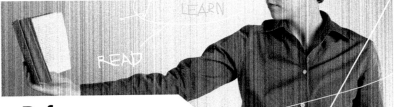

References

1. *Prevention of Low Back Pain.* Shelby County Health System. www.myrtue.org. 22 January 2000.

2. Rolf, Ida P. *Rolfing: Reestablishing the Natural Alignment and Structural Integration of the Human Body.* Rochester: Healing Arts Press, 1989.

3. *Back and Neck Care Guide.* McKinley Health Center, University of Illinois. 8 February 2000. www.uiuc.edu.departments/mckinley/health-info/fitness/back. 3 March 2000.

4. Muscolino, Joseph E. *Electronic Communication.* June 2003.

7 *Bending*

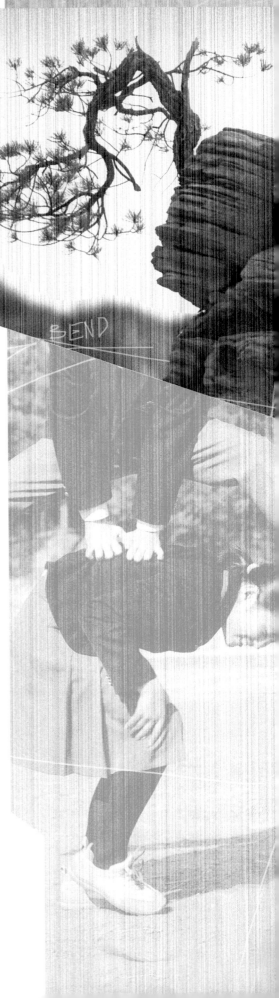

Introduction

Whether standing or sitting, bending is a function that, as a manual therapist, you constantly use. There is absolutely no way to avoid bending, primarily because manual therapy requires you to transfer your work from a vertical position to a horizontal one. An obvious example is standing or sitting (vertically) while working with a client who is lying (horizontally). Of course, you can also stand or sit while working on a client who is seated. In this case, although your client is also vertical, you still must bend in order to reach them.

Identifying your false hip joints, bending from your true hip joints, counterbalancing your upper body and pelvis and leg alignment will be our focus in this chapter. Attention will be given to keeping your body, especially your back, safe from discomfort and injury while bending.

Before you read this chapter…

How often do you bend on a daily basis?

○ *almost always*
○ *sometimes*
○ *not very often*
○ *other_____*

What parts of your body are you most aware of when bending?

○ *head and neck*
○ *shoulders and upper back*
○ *pelvis and legs*
○ *other_____*

What parts of your body are you least aware of when bending?

○ *head and neck*
○ *shoulders and upper back*
○ *pelvis and legs*
○ *other_____*

Describe 5 daily activities that involve bending.

1. _____
2. _____
3. _____
4. _____
5. _____

Describe an everyday activity involving bending that you do with ease and comfort.

_____

_____

Describe an everyday activity involving bending that you do with difficulty or discomfort.

_____

_____

How comfortable are you bending on an everyday basis?

○ *always*
○ *mostly*
○ *sometimes*
○ *very seldom*

Your false hip joints

Bending, as a movement, is not a problem when done primarily with the hip joints. The problem begins when the movement of bending is made mainly with the spine. As mentioned previously, bending forward from the low back is one of three factors commonly seen in people with low back pain. For many therapists, bending from the back is a habitual pattern, one that is used over and over again. This repetitive pattern, due in part to a downward focus, leads to vertebral strain over time, causing bending to be an uncomfortable function to perform. Understanding the difference between your "true hip joints" and "false hip joints" will make bending more comfortable, causing less strain to your back.

Your false hip joints are the areas in your spine where you *habitually* bend from, typically, from the cervical or from the lumbar spine. (7.1) Constantly bending from your spine causes a chronic lengthening in the back muscles and an overuse of the vertebral discs, joints and ligaments.[1] Your back and spine cannot endure this kind of strain and will, in the long run, suffer.

The following *Self-observation* lesson will help you recognize where in your back you tend to bend from. During the lesson, identify your false hip joints and see if this place corresponds to an area of your back that is typically tired or sore after your treatments.

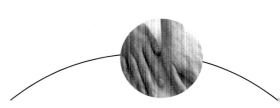

Practice tip 7.1

Bending repetitively from the low back leaves many manual therapists with the inability to fully extend. As mentioned in Chapter 6, these two activities, frequent flexion (bending forward at the waist) and the inability to fully extend (bend backwards) are two of three factors commonly seen in people with low back pain. If you are constantly bending throughout your session, balance your flexion with extension. Take time to, slowly and gently, bend backward throughout your day.

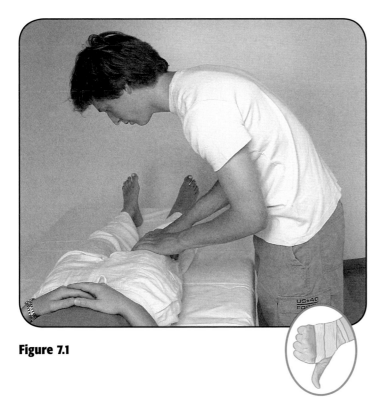

Figure 7.1

Identifying your false hip joints

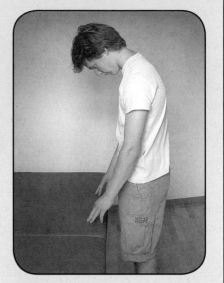

Stand next to your table, vertically aligned, using the tripods of your feet and in a parallel stance. Reach your hands toward your table, bending forward using your neck, upper back and shoulders. (7.2)

Tip This movement will feel like you are collapsing into your upper back.

Notice how the muscles in your neck, upper back and shoulders feel as you make this movement.
Can you feel effort in your neck?
Can you easily reach your arms toward your table?

Notice if bending in this manner feels familiar to you.
Would you consider your neck, upper back and shoulders to be your false hip joints?

Rest.

Figure 7.2

Stand again as before, and reach your hands toward your table, this time bending from your mid back. Your shoulders will also be involved in this movement, but try to initiate the bending from the middle of your back. (7.3)

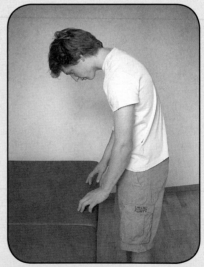

Tip This movement will feel like you are curving your mid-back into a "C".

Notice how your chest and rib cage feel as you make this movement.
How does it affect your breathing?
Can you easily reach your arms toward your table?

Notice if bending in this manner feels familiar to you.
Would you consider your mid-back to be your false hip joints?

Rest.

Finally, stand as before, and reach your hands toward your table, bending from your low back. Your upper and mid-back will bend too, but initiate the bending from your lower back. (7.4)

Figure 7.3

continued

Tip This movement will feel as if you are curving your low back concavely.

Notice in what direction your pelvis moves when you bend from your low back.
Does your pelvis tilt forward or backward?
How does your back feel when bending this way?
Can you easily reach your arms toward your table?

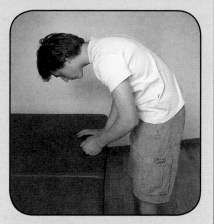

Figure 7.4

Notice if bending in this manner feels familiar to you.
Would you consider your lower back to be your false hip joints?

Rest.

Now that you have identified your false hip joints, you can be more aware when you are using them. The next *Self-observation* lesson will teach you how to bend using your true hip joints, giving you a healthier alternative to bending from your back.

Self-feedback
What part of your back did you identify as your false hip joints?

_____

Is this part of your back a place where you experience strain?

_____

What part of your back, when bending, felt unfamiliar?

_____

Something to think about...

How often do you bend during a typical session?

_____

_____

Where do you tend to bend from?

_____

_____

How comfortable are you bending?

_____

_____

Do you try to avoid bending? If so, why and what do you do instead?

_____

_____

_____

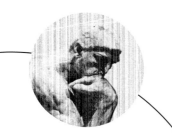

Your true hip joints

The hip joint is located where the femur meets the pelvis structure. The best way to experience its movement is to either stand or sit and simply lift your leg. Putting your fingers in the crease of your leg and pelvis will help you feel the actual articulation of the joint. An interesting fact to note is the hip joints are the sole connecting points between your entire upper body and legs. Hence, it is no surprise that the ball and socket joint of the hip is the strongest and one of the most stable in your body.

When bending from your true hip joints, you recruit the powerful muscles of your pelvis and legs. (7.5) These muscles, along with the strong and stable ball and socket joints of your hips, can easily support your weight and facilitate your bending movements. This relieves the muscular effort of your back and decreases spinal stress.

Consider this

Just how strong are ball and socket joints? Well, the folks who built Stonehenge knew. Stonehenge (3100-1550 BC) is a megalithic monument on Salisbury Plain in Wiltshire, England. Massive stones, weighing as much as 26 tons, were placed on top of each other, stabilized only by ball and socket joints. Each vertical stone has a ball and each horizontal a socket. [3] *(7.6.)*

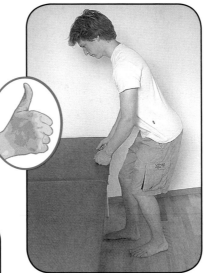

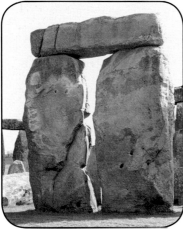

Figure 7.6

Figure 7.5

Bending from your true hip joints requires you to bend from your knees and ankles as well. This increases your flexibility and stability. Bending from your hip joints without the use of your knees and ankles causes tremendous strain on your back. In this case, the weight of your upper body is not counterbalanced with the weight of your pelvis, causing your upper body's weight to be suspended out in front of you. Take a few minutes to explore the following:

Bend forward using only your hip joints, keep your knees and ankles straight.

Notice how bending in this manner feels.

Now bend forward using your hip joints, knees and ankles.

Can you feel the difference?

Note: If you experience pain in your knees when bending with your hips, knees and ankles, find a way that feels more comfortable. Though bending from the hip joints, knees and ankles is healthier for the back, it requires a certain amount of strength in these areas.

Bending from your true hip joints

Stand next to your table, vertically aligned, using the tripods of your feet and in a parallel stance. Reach your hands toward your table and bend using your hip joints, knees and ankles. As you bend your upper body forward, bend your knees and ankles, keeping your upper, mid and low back in a neutral position. (7.7)

Tip It is common to hyperextend or exaggerate the lumbar curve when bending from the hip joints, but your low back should remain in a neutral position as you bend.

Continue to reach toward your table several times, bending from your hip joints. If you find that you begin to bend from your spine, stop the bending, bringing your back into a neutral position again. Each time you bend, become clearer that you are bending from your true hip joints and not your false ones.

Notice the movement you have in your upper body when bending from your hip joints.
Do you sense ease of movement in your arms?
Do you sense ease of movement in your shoulders and neck?
Does your back feel relaxed?

Rest.

Stand this time in a one-foot forward stance. Reach toward your table, bending from your hip joints. Even though you are using a different stance, continue to bend both knees and ankles. (7.8)

Tip The tendency in this stance is to only bend the front knee - be sure to bend both.

Notice the movement you have in your upper body in this stance.
Do you sense ease of movement in your arms?
Do you sense ease of movement in your shoulders and neck?
Does your back feel relaxed?

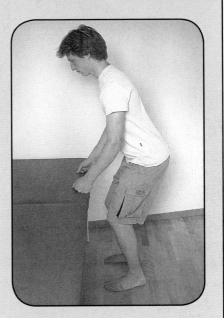

Figure 7.7

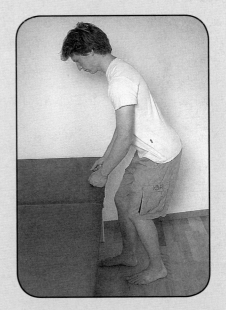

Figure 7.8

continued

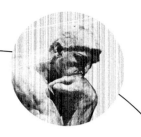

Consider this

Your vertebral column, or spine, has three main regions and consists of twenty-four verte-brae. There are seven cervical (neck), twelve thoracic (mid-back) and five lumbar (low back). Your sacrum and coccyx (tailbone) are also part of your spine, having fused vertebrae. Out of the three regions, your cervical spine has the most range of motion, and allows for the movement of your head. Your thoracic spine articulates with your twelve ribs, has the least amount of mobility, and helps to stabilize your rib cage. Finally, your lumbar spine is considerably larger and helps to support your body's weight. [2]

Continue to reach toward your table, switching between this and a parallel stance. Take as much time as you need to become comfortable with bending from your hip joints. Don't worry if you feel yourself bending from your back, just notice it and continue. Over time, bending from your hip joints will become natural to you.

Bending from your hip joints liberates your spine and back. Instead of recruiting all its structures for bending, the spine and back muscles can facilitate the fine and skillful work of your therapy, leaving the hard work of bending to the capable true hip joints.

Self-feedback
Compare the differences between bending with your false hip joints and with your true hip joints.

_____

_____

How can bending with your true hip joints improve the quality of your touch?

_____

_____

How can bending with your true hip joints improve the overall quality of your body mechanics?

_____

_____

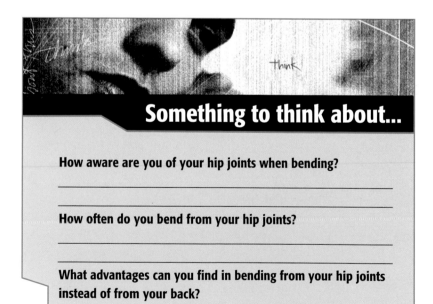

Something to think about...

How aware are you of your hip joints when bending?

_____

How often do you bend from your hip joints?

_____

What advantages can you find in bending from your hip joints instead of from your back?

_____

_____

Counterbalance

As you have experienced in the last lesson, when bending from your hip joints, it is important to bend your knees and ankles. With this movement, you are able to counterbalance the weight of your upper body with the weight of your pelvis. Counterbalancing your body's weight keeps your center of gravity over your legs and feet.[4] With this kind of balance, you maintain a sense of self-support (discussed in upcoming chapters) and can freely move and bend from your hip joints, leaving your back, shoulders, arms and hands free to facilitate your manual therapy.

There are some excellent examples of counterbalance found in the world of sports, such as surfing and mountain biking. Not only do surfers live to ride the perfect wave, they also know a thing or two about bending and counterbalance. Look at how a surfer rides his board and you will see he bends from his hip joints, knees and ankles, and counterbalances the weight of his upper body and pelvis. Bending from his hip joints allows his upper body to remain flexible and free to move, while counterbalancing allows him to remain stable on his feet and board. (7.9)

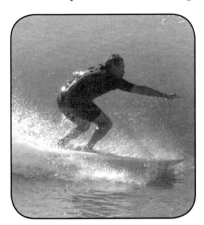

Figure 7.9

Mountain bikers also have the art of bending and counterbalance down to a science. In order to stay on her bike, a mountain biker must bend from the hip joints, knees and ankles and, at the same time, counterbalance the weight of her pelvis and upper body while maneuvering her bike over difficult terrain. (7.10)

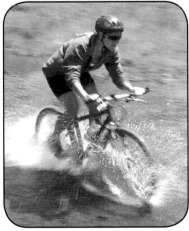

Figure 7.10

These two sports show clear examples of counterbalance. For your purpose as a therapist, you will not make such inordinate movements, but the concepts remain the same. Your use of counterbalance may be much more subtle, but is as important to producing a quality outcome, the comfort and ease of movement.

The following *Self-observation* lesson will help clarify the concept of counterbalance.

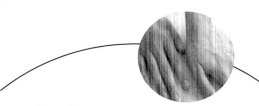

Practice tip 7.2

How hip are you? Stand and point to where you think your hip joints are. Where are you pointing? Are you pointing to the outside of your hips, where your greater trochanter is? Or are you pointing to the inside, toward the crease of your pelvis and leg? If you are pointing to the inside of your hips, congratulations! You are right, your hip joints are actually inside, where your pelvis and leg form a crease.

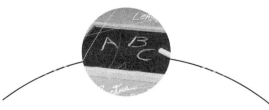

Client education tip 7.1

Like many of us, our clients also bend from the back, using the spine instead of the hip joints. If you have a client with chronic back pain, ask him or her to slowly bend forward, watching for movement in the spine and hip joints. If your client primarily bends from somewhere in the spine, point this out, explaining the difference between bending from the back and bending from the hip joints. If appropriate, slowly lead your client through the Self-observation 7.2 lesson.

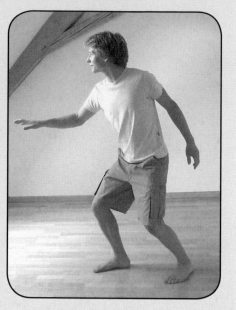

The art of counterbalance

Stand in front of a mirror and pretend that you are surfing, imagining that you are on a surfboard and riding a big wave. (7.11)

Notice how you instinctively stand.
Are you bending from your hip joints?
Are you counterbalancing your upper body and pelvis?
Where do you intuitively place your feet?

If you were not bending from your hip joints and counterbalancing before, do it now, feeling how these concepts increase your stability.

Rest.

Stand next to your table, vertically aligned, using the tripods of your feet and in a comfortable stance. Begin to reach toward your table, bending from your hip joints, knees and ankles, and counterbalancing your upper body and pelvis. (7.12)

Figure 7.11

Tip Your spine should be in a neutral position, with no effort felt in your back.

Notice how your back responds to this movement.
Can you sense less effort in your back muscles?
Can you sense less effort in your shoulders and arms?
Can you move your head freely?
Can you breathe freely?

Rest.

Stand, as before, next to your table. Reach toward your table but this time, bend with your back without counterbalancing your pelvis and upper body. (7.13)

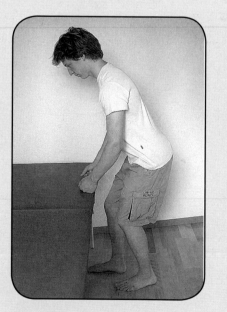

Figure 7.12

Notice the difference between how you are bending now and how you were bending with your hip joints before.
Can you sense more effort in your back muscles?
Can you sense more effort in your shoulders and arms?

continued

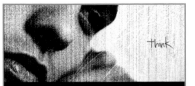

Can you move your head freely?
Can you breathe freely?

Rest.

Stand as before. Once more begin to reach toward your table, bending from your hip joints, knees and ankles, and counterbalancing your pelvis and upper body.

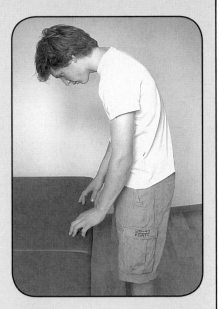

Notice again the difference between bending with counterbalance and bending from your back, as before.

Figure 7.13

What differences do you feel in your back?
What differences do you sense in your shoulders and arms?
What differences do you sense in your body in general?

Counterbalance is the secret to effortless bending. Using your hip joints is crucial, but using them in combination with counterbalance is the final key to effective and comfortable bending.

Self-feedback
How does the use of counterbalance influence the comfort of your bending?

_____

_____

Can you feel the advantages of counterbalancing?

_____

_____

In what other areas of your life can you imagine using this concept?

_____

_____

Something to think about...

Can you think of some activities in which you have successfully applied the concept of counterbalance?

_____

_____

What sports, besides surfing and mountain biking, employ the concept of counterbalance?

_____

_____

What are the advantages of using counterbalance when bending?

_____

_____

_____

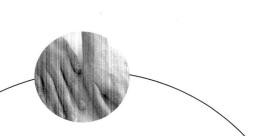

Practice tip 7.3

If you are finding it difficult to counterbalance your pelvis with your upper body, try imagining a string attached to your tailbone. As you bend, the string gently pulls your pelvis backward, as your head leans forward. The movement of the pelvis is subtle, but once you become more aware of it, counterbalancing will become more natural to you.

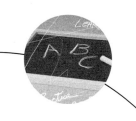

Client education tip 7.2

If you have a client who is a surfer, skateboarder and/or snowboarder, and is experiencing back pain, explain and show him or her the concept of counterbalance. They may already know the concept in theory, but may not be putting it into practice.

Leg alignment

One thing you may have noticed when considering the different examples of bending and counterbalance presented, is that each athlete depends on the legs for support. In order for the legs to effectively support the weight of the body, the joints of the legs must stay in relative alignment with each other. This increases skeletal support and protects the joints from strain.

As a therapist, keep this principle in mind as well. Be attentive to the placement of your feet in relation to your knees and hip joints. (7.14) If you stand with your feet wide apart, make sure you can maintain your knee and foot alignment. (7.15) If not, stand with your feet closer together.

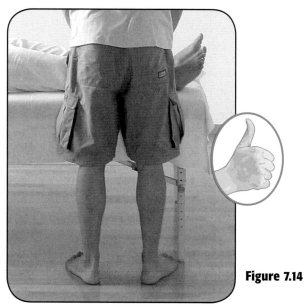

Figure 7.14

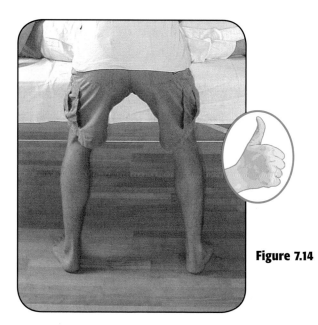

Figure 7.14

Bending while sitting

It is crucial to realize that bending from the hip joints is as important when sitting as it is when standing. Many manual therapists find themselves bending from the back when reaching forward, for example, to push and pull when working in a seated position. Bending from your hip joints decreases the strain and fatigue often felt when working in a seated position. Your shoulders, arms and hands are free to move, while your legs and feet support the weight of your body.

The following *Self-exploration* lesson will help guide you through this process.

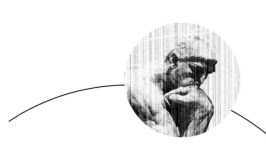

Consider this

The stance of a sumo wrestler is a great example of bending, counterbalance and alignment. To efficiently support his weight, he must stand with proper alignment, with his knees over his feet. With this stance, he is using the strength of his skeleton and the strong muscles of his lower body to support his massive size.[5] *(7.16)*

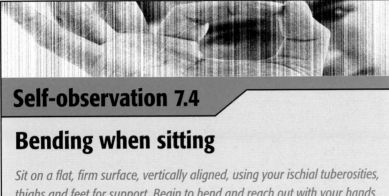

Self-observation 7.4

Bending when sitting

Sit on a flat, firm surface, vertically aligned, using your ischial tuberosities, thighs and feet for support. Begin to bend and reach out with your hands as if beginning to work with a client.

Notice where you begin to bend from.
Do you start bending from your mid or upper back?
Do you bend from your neck?

Now imagine there is a table just in front of your knees. Bend forward to put your nose on the table. (7.17)

Notice how you make this movement.
Do you bend from you neck?
Do you bend from somewhere in your back?

Rest.

Sit as before. Begin to make the above movement again, but this time bend forward using

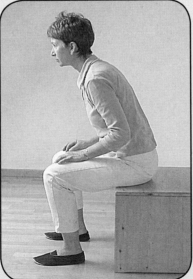

Figure 7.17

your hip joints to bring your nose closer the table. Keep your back, neck and head in a neutral position as you bend forward.

continued

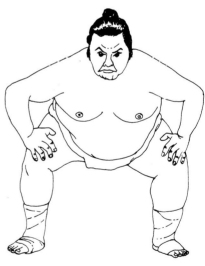

Figure 7.16

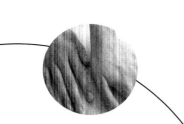

Practice tip 7.4

Often, improper alignment is the cause of knee and ankle strain. Take a few minutes each day to stand like a sumo. Stand in front of a mirror to check your alignment or ask a friend to do so. This will help reinforce the importance of proper alignment and increase the muscular tone in your legs.

Rest.

Sit as before, and bend forward once again using your hip joints.

Notice what you sense in your legs and feet.
Do you sense how your legs and feet can support you? Do you sense the weight increasing in your feet as you bend forward?

Tip Your legs and feet play important roles in supporting your weight and movement forward.

Continue to bend from your hip joints, bringing your nose closer to the imaginary table in front of your knees. (7.18)

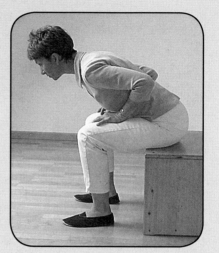

Figure 7.18

How does your back, neck and head feel bending in this way?

Stop bending from your hip joints and bend forward using your back or neck. Compare how bending in this way feels to bending forward using your hip joints.

Do you sense more or less effort in your neck and back, bending in this manner?

Now return to bending forward using your hip joints.

Rest.

This time sit, as before, facing your therapy table. Reach with your hands toward your table and bend forward using your hip joints. (7.19) *Keep your back, neck and head in a neutral position.*

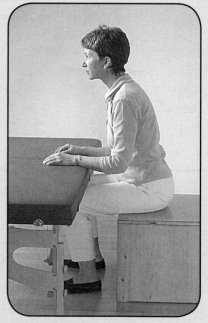

Figure 7.19

continued

Notice the freedom of movement you have in your upper body when bending from your hip joints.
Do you have a sense of comfort and ease in your shoulders, arms and hands?
Do you have a sense of comfort and ease in your neck and back?

Notice the support your legs and feet give when bending in this manner.
Do you sense how your legs and feet support your weight?

For a moment, reach toward your table, bending forward using your back. (7.20)

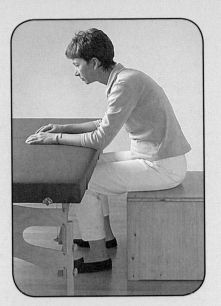

Figure 7.20

Notice the response in your upper body when bending in this manner.
Do you feel a lack of movement in your shoulders, arms and hands?
Do you sense an increase of muscular tension in your neck and back?
How does this style of bending affect your breathing?

Notice the lack of support in your legs and feet when bending in this manner.
Do you sense how your legs and feet are less able to support your weight?

Now return to bending from your hip joints and begin to reach your hands toward the right side of your table. (7.21)

Tip As you bend to the right, your left foot can help assist the movement by pressing into the floor and directing your movement to the right.

Do you feel your weight shift a bit to your right side?

Now reach toward the left side of your table, bending from your hip joints.

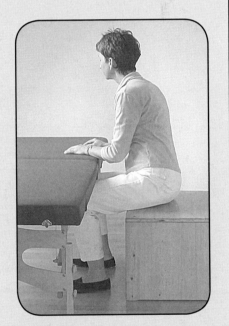

Figure 7.21

Tip As you bend to the left, your right foot can help assist the movement by pressing into the floor and directing your moment to the left.

Do you feel your weight shift a bit to your left side?

continued

Begin to alternate, reaching toward one side of your table and then toward the other side. Continue to make these movements until they feel comfortable to you.

Rest.

When sitting, bend from your hip joints and allow your legs and feet to support you. This will keep your back, neck and head free from strain and discomfort, and your shoulders, arms and hands free to move with ease.

Self-feedback

Is the concept of bending from your hip joints while sitting new to you? If so, what are your thoughts about it?

_____

_____

_____

_____

What are the advantages of bending from your hip joints while sitting? _____

_____

_____

_____

_____

_____

How can you incorporate this concept into other daily sitting activities? _____

_____

_____

_____

Now that you've read this chapter...

How aware are you now of your bending habits?
- ○ *almost always*
- ○ *sometimes*
- ○ *not very often*
- ○ *other_____*

When bending, what parts of your body are you now most aware of?
- ○ *neck and shoulders*
- ○ *arms and hands*
- ○ *pelvis and legs*
- ○ *other_____*

When bending, what parts of your body are you still not aware of?
- ○ *neck and shoulders*
- ○ *arms and hands*
- ○ *pelvis and legs*
- ○ *other_____*

Describe 4 concepts that make bending more dynamic.

1. _____

2. _____

3. _____

4. _____

Describe an aspect of bending that feels easy and comfortable.

_____

_____

Describe an aspect of bending that you do not feel comfortable with yet.

_____

_____

How comfortable are you now bending?
- ○ *completely*
- ○ *mostly*
- ○ *a little*
- ○ *not very*

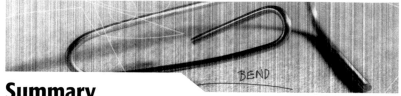

Summary

In this chapter, you have learned how to identify your false hip joints and explored how to bend from your true hip joints when standing and sitting. You have learned about the concept of counterbalance and how to use it with regard to your upper body and pelvis. The importance of leg alignment was also discussed. Here's a review of the concepts learned in the chapter:

For many therapists, bending from the spine is a habitual pattern, leading to vertebral strain. Your **false hip joints** are the areas in your spine where you habitually bend from. The **true hip joints** are the sole connecting points between your entire upper body and legs, and are the strongest and one of the most stable joints in your body. When used for bending, your hip joints can easily support your weight and facilitate your movements, relieving muscular effort and decreasing spinal stress. **Counterbalancing** your upper body and pelvis keeps your center of gravity over your legs and feet. With this kind of balance, you can bend from your hip, knee and ankle joints, leaving your back, shoulders, arms and hands free to facilitate your manual therapy. **Leg alignment** increases skeletal support and protects the joints from strain.

When sitting to work, bend from your hip joints and allow your legs and feet to support you. This will keep your back, neck and head free from strain and discomfort, and your shoulders, arms and hands free to move with ease.

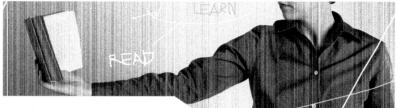

References

1. Back Pain: *Common and Uncommon Causes.* Mayo Foundation for Medical Education and Research. 2000. www.mayohealth.org. 22 January 2000.

2. Goldstein, Jeffrey. *Understanding How the Back Works.* Back Pain Health Center. 2002. www.health.yahoo.com/health/centers/back_pain. 22 May 2003.

3. Stonehenge. *Britannica Ready Reference.* Encyclopedia Britannica, Inc. 2001.

4. Haller, Jeff. *Feldenkrais Professional Training Program.* Maui, Hawaii, 1994.

5. Mina, Hall. *The Big Book of Sumo.* Berkeley: Stone Bridge Press, 1998.

8 Lifting

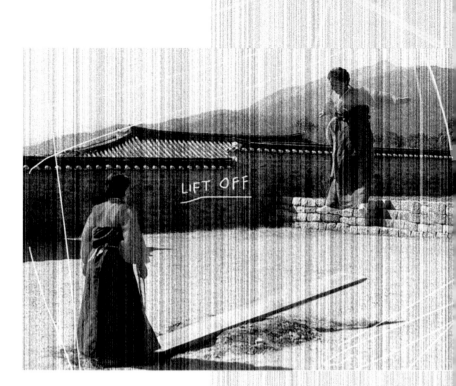

Introduction

The American Journal of Public Health ranked health care therapists 8th on a list of the top 10 jobs with the highest prevalence of low back pain due to an injury at work - improper lifting is said to be one of the main reasons low back pain occurs.[1]

Lifting, like bending, is unavoidable in manual therapy and even though it has a bad reputation for causing discomfort and injury, can be done safely and comfortably. Whether you lift frequently throughout your treatments or just occasionally, learning how to lift properly will protect your back from unnecessary stress and possible injury.

In this chapter, you will learn and experience the importance of getting close to the weight you are lifting, using the power of your lower body and facing the proper direction. You will also learn how to reduce stress in your back and upper body by lifting, holding and moving a weight using the support of your lower body. Once you implement these key concepts, you will lift with confidence.

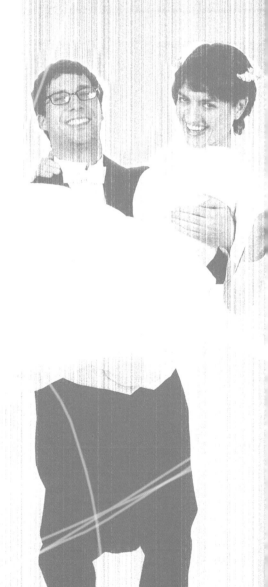

Before you read this chapter...

How often do you lift on a daily basis?
- ○ *almost always*
- ○ *sometimes*
- ○ *not very often*
- ○ *other_____*

What parts of your body are you most aware of when lifting?
- ○ *head and neck*
- ○ *shoulders and upper back*
- ○ *pelvis and legs*
- ○ *other_____*

What parts of your body are you least aware of when lifting?
- ○ *head and neck*
- ○ *shoulders and upper back*
- ○ *pelvis and legs*
- ○ *other_____*

Describe 5 lifting habits that you are aware of on a daily basis.
(e.g., lifting with your legs)

1. _____
2. _____
3. _____
4. _____
5. _____

Describe an everyday activity involving lifting that you do with ease and comfort.

_____
_____

Describe an everyday activity involving lifting that you do with difficulty or discomfort.

_____
_____

How comfortable are you lifting on an everyday basis?
- ○ *completely*
- ○ *mostly*
- ○ *a little*
- ○ *not at all*

Get close

When lifting, for example, the head, get as close to your client as possible. (8.1) If you find that leaning on your table is helpful for leverage, do so without losing your balance and control. If needed, ask your client to come closer to you, decreasing the space between you and the weight. Getting as close as possible will decrease the pressure on your spine and minimize your risk for injury.

A common mistake made is lifting weight that is too far from the body, for example, standing at arm's length when lifting a client's leg or head. (8.2) When doing so, you must reach and then lift, leaning toward the weight and putting a tremendous strain on the muscles and vertebrae of your back. This style of lifting also requires the muscles of your arms and shoulders to work hard, first to reach the weight and then to lift it.

Getting as close as possible, no matter the amount of weight, is one of the simplest and smartest rules of proper lifting. [?]

The following *Self-observation* lesson will assist you in exploring this concept.

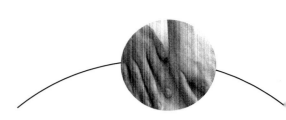

Practice tip 8.1

The next time you are lifting a client's leg, notice how far you are standing from your table. If you are standing several inches away, notice how heavy his/her leg feels. Move closer to your table and again, notice the sense of weight. What distance makes the leg feel lighter?

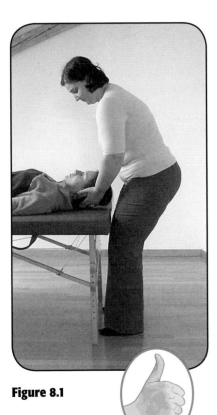

Figure 8.1

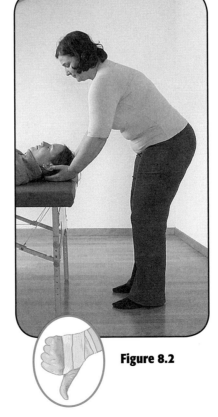

Figure 8.2

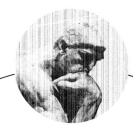

Consider this

Lifting an object weighing 10 pounds at arm's length, puts 150 pounds of force on the back. An object weighing 86 pounds puts over 700 pounds of force on the discs in the lower back. [3]

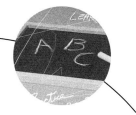

Client education tip 8.1

Standing close when lifting is a tip all of your clients can benefit from. Clients who frequently bend and pick up children, for example, can be reminded to stand close to the child before lifting.

Self-observation 8.1

Lifting from far and near

Place a heavy book, for example, a telephone book, on the end of your table. Stand a full arm's length away, lift the book with both hands and hold it up for a few seconds. (8.3)

Sense the muscular effort that you are using.
Can you feel the strain this distance puts on your neck, shoulders and back?

Sense how heavy the book feels.
Does it feel heavier than it actually is?

Notice your breathing.
Can you breathe comfortably while lifting from this distance?

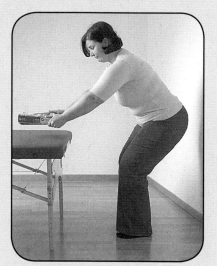

Figure 8.3

Rest.

Now stand a few inches away and lift the book with both hands. (8.4)

Sense the amount of muscular effort you are using at this distance.
Has the muscular effort decreased in your neck, shoulders and back?

Sense how heavy the book feels.
Is it lighter or heavier than it was before?

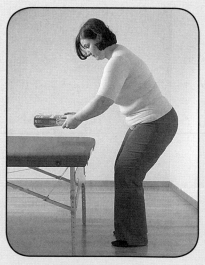

Figure 8.4

continued

Notice your breathing.
Can you breathe more comfortably?

Rest.

Now stand as close to your table as possible and lift the book with both hands.(8.5)

Sense the amount of muscular effort you are using standing close.

Has the muscular effort further decreased in your neck, shoulders and back?

Sense how heavy the book feels.
Is it lighter than it was before?

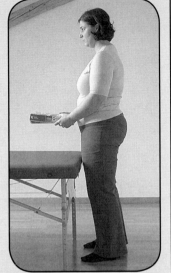

Figure 8.5

Notice your breathing.
Can you breathe more comfortably?

Become aware of the distance between you and your client when lifting, and lift from a close proximity. This gives you a leverage advantage, decreases muscular work and increases your comfort and effectiveness.

Self-feedback
How heavy did the object feel when standing and lifting: at arm's length, a few inches away and in close proximity?

_____

_____

What was the difference regarding muscular effort when lifting from these three distances?

_____

_____

What are the advantages of standing close when lifting?

_____

_____

_____

_____

Something to think about...

How many times a day do you lift something up? (e.g., coffee cup, a pet, the newspaper)

_____

_____

How often do you lift during a typical session?

_____

_____

At what distance do you tend to stand when lifting a client's leg or head?

_____

_____

Do you feel comfortable standing close to your table when lifting? Explain.

_____

_____

_____

_____

Face it

Another common error made is lifting while in a rotated stance. This is said to be one of the leading causes of low back injuries.[4] When your body is rotated while lifting, the vertebrae, discs and soft tissue of your back are under significant pressure and your overall stability is compromised. Lifting any amount of weight in rotation, no matter how light, puts tremendous strain on your body.

A tendency for most manual therapists is to lift, for example, a client's leg while standing in a rotated position, facing the intended direction of movement, instead of directly facing the weight itself. (8.6) In this situation, the therapist's lower body is directed toward the leg, while her upper body is rotated toward the head of the table. This style of lifting compromises the therapist's alignment, stressing the muscles and joints of the back, shoulders and arms.

Face the weight to keep your body in proper alignment, eliminate rotation and decrease your strain and effort. Keep your feet, pelvis and upper body directed toward the weight to insure you are facing it without rotation. (8.7)

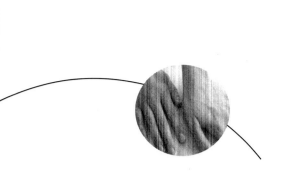
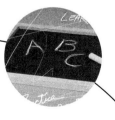
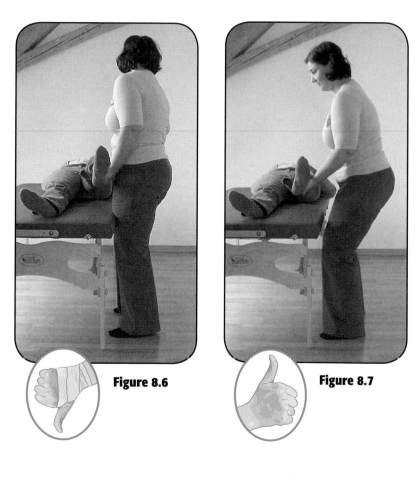

Figure 8.6

Figure 8.7

Let your legs lift it

"Lift with your legs, not your back" is a well-known phrase used when discussing the everyday body mechanics of lifting. It is excellent advice and should be applied to the body mechanics of manual therapy as well.

Lifting with your legs means you are using the power of your lower body to lift the weight. Keep your spine vertically aligned, bend from your hip joints, knees and ankles, and use the power of your legs, instead of bending from your back and putting strain on your spine and upper body. (8.8) This saves your low back and upper body from undue strain and allows the larger and stronger muscles of your lower body to do the work.

Therapists often lift by using only their upper body, which causes muscle fatigue and stress. (8.9) The secret to easier lifting is: *before* you begin to lift the weight, bend from your hip joints, knees and ankles. (8.10) *As you lift* the weight, press your feet into the floor and straighten your legs, without locking your knees. (8.11) (Basically, you are raising *your* body to raise the weight.) *To lower* the weight, bend your hip joints, knees and ankles, and return to your original starting position. (8.12) Lift in this manner to allow your back to remain vertical and reduce excessive muscular effort in your shoulders, arms and hands. Your upper body facilitates the lifting, while the strong muscles of your legs do the hard work!

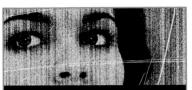

Something to think about...

Do you tend to lift your client's limbs from a rotated position? Explain.

_____

_____

Do you tend to lift more from the left or right side of your table? Explain.

_____

_____

What are the advantages of facing the weight while lifting?

_____

_____

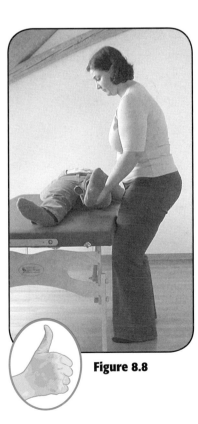

Figure 8.8

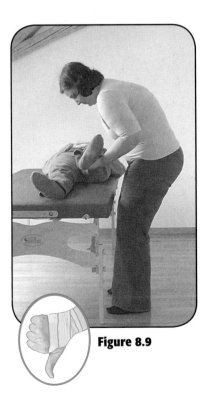

Figure 8.9

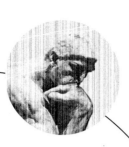

Consider this

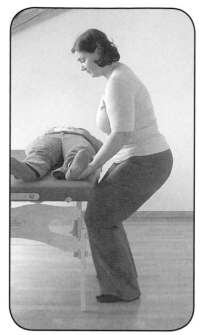

Figure 8.10

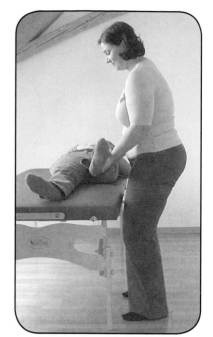

Figure 8.11

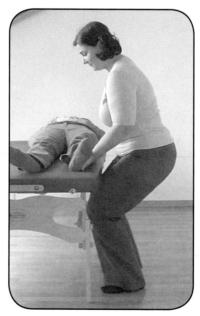

Figure 8.12

Life after lifting

Once you have lifted a weight, for example, a client's leg, you will probably want to move it. If so, there are two choices, both of which will keep your back safe from injury. If not, simply remain in your position.

The first choice is to remain in your original lifting position. (8.13) From this position you can take side-steps while facing the weight, moving the client's leg in the direction of the head or foot of the table. (8.14) Your feet should be in a parallel stance and your legs in good alignment.

The second choice is to reposition yourself while holding the weight. This means *after* you have lifted the leg, reposition yourself to fully face the intended direction of movement, e.g., the head of the table. (8.15) Your feet should be in a one-foot forward stance and your legs in a good alignment. If you need to make a large movement, take steps forward or back.

When holding the weight, let your lower body support it by maintaining good leg alignment and using the tripods of your feet. This will allow your upper body to facilitate the holding, without excessive muscular effort. However, never hold a weight longer than is comfortable - always rest when needed. If you cannot comfortably

Something to think about...

Is lifting with your legs a concept you have heard before? Explain.

_____

_____

When working, do you tend to lift with your legs or your back? Explain.

_____

_____

Are you comfortable when lifting? If not, why?

_____

_____

What are the advantages of lifting with your legs?

_____

_____

_____

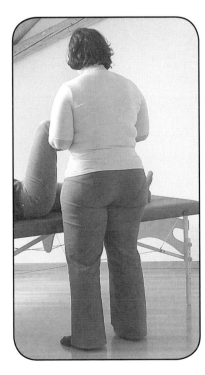

Figure 8.13

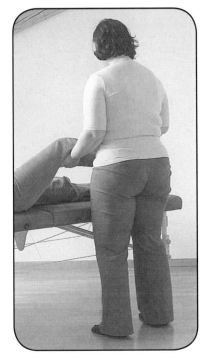

Figure 8.14

hold the weight, chances are you are standing too far away and/or the weight is too heavy. If either or both is the case, put the weight down, stand closer and/or ask your client to assist in the lifting, holding and moving process.

The following *Partner practice* lesson will help you experience the two choices of lifting and moving we have just discussed.

Practice tip 8.3

Avoid reaching across the mid-line of your table to lift. Reaching and lifting across the mid-line compromises the alignment of the spine and increases the chance of strain and injury. Take the time to walk around your table, lifting from a close and comfortable proximity.

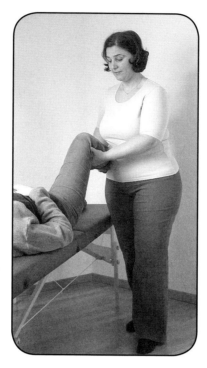

Figure 8.15

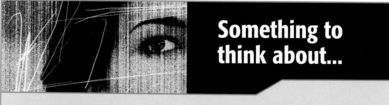

Something to think about...

What are some of the reasons you lift during a session?

_____

_____

Are there times when you could ask your client for more help with lifting? If so, when?

_____

_____

Do you feel comfortable asking for help when lifting? If not, why?

_____

_____

How often do you lift, hold and move during a session?

_____

_____

Lifting, holding and moving

Ask your partner to lie down on his or her back, and stand beside your table, facing the lower leg. Make sure your entire body, including your feet, faces the leg. Keeping your back in a neutral position, slowly begin to bend from your hip joints, knees and ankles. Once your hands and arms are parallel with the leg, hold it with both hands and begin to lift your partner's leg by straightening your legs. Allow your partner's leg to bend at the knee. Repeat this sequence of movements a few times until you feel comfortable with it. (8.16)

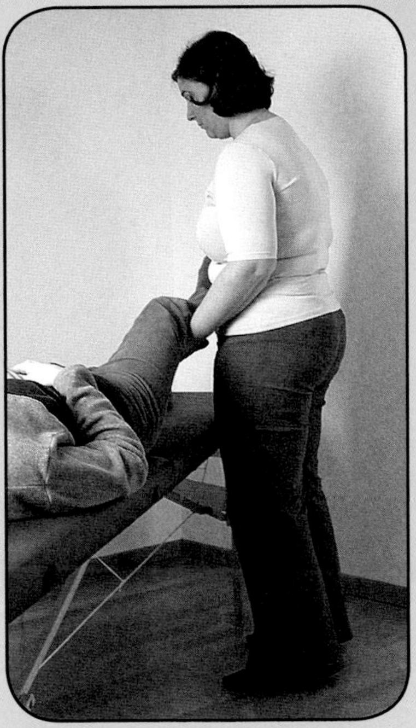

Tip This style of lifting allows you to keep your shoulders and arms relaxed while holding your partner's leg. Let your shoulders remain in a neutral and comfortable position, not held up and/or tense. Allow your elbows to rest comfortably by your sides, not held out in space.

Figure 8.16

Notice what you sense in your legs.
Can you sense your feet pressing into the floor as you straighten your legs?
Are your legs able to support the lifting?

Notice what you sense in your upper body.
Are you able to keep your back in a neutral position?
Are you able to let your legs lift, and your back, shoulders and arms relax?

Rest.

Begin to lift again, as before. As you begin to lift, press your feet into the floor while straightening your legs. Lift and lower your partner's leg in this manner a few times.

Tip By pressing your feet into the floor and straightening your legs, you are using the strength and power of your lower body to lift your partner's leg. This allows your upper body to relax and comfortably facilitate the lifting without strain and effort.

Notice the effectiveness of your lifting now.
By pressing your feet, can you sense more strength in your legs?
Are you able to use less effort in your upper body?
Is the lifting easier now?

Rest.

continued

In the same manner as before, lift your partner's leg, holding it up. Remain facing the leg, with your feet in a parallel stance. Slowly begin to move your partner's knee in the direction of his or her chest. (8.17) Be sure to keep your back, shoulders and arms as relaxed as possible.

Try making a larger movement by taking a few steps in the direction of the head of the table. Next, try a larger movement toward the foot of the table by taking a few steps in that direction.

Notice how this technique affects the quality of your lifting and movement.

Can you maintain your vertical alignment when taking side-steps?
Are your legs able to do the work of the movement?
Are you able to reduce the muscular effort in your upper body?

Rest.

As before, lift your partner's leg. This time before you move the knee, reposition yourself by turning your feet and body so you are facing the head of the table. (8.18) Before you start to move, be sure that your body is not rotated. Your feet should now be in a one-foot forward stance.

Slowly begin to move your partner's leg, bringing the knee toward the chest and then back to its neutral position. (8.19) When you are ready to return the leg to the table, first reposition yourself to face the leg, and then lower it down. Continue to lift, hold and move your partner's leg in this manner a few times until you feel comfortable with it.

Tip Take as many steps as needed to advance your entire body in the direction of the movement. This will help maintain your vertical alignment, keep you close to the weight and reduce the muscular effort and strain in your upper body.

Notice how this technique affects the quality of your lifting and movement.

When moving the leg, can you maintain your vertical alignment?
Are your legs able to do the work of the movement?
Are you able to reduce the muscular effort in your back, shoulders and arms?

Rest.

Lifting, holding and moving weight utilizing these techniques will protect your body from injury. While the strong muscles and joints of your legs support and move the weight, your back, shoulders and arms can remain comfortable and relaxed.

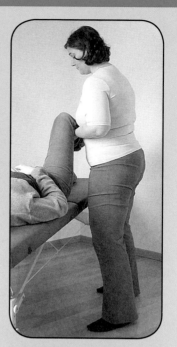

Figure 8.17

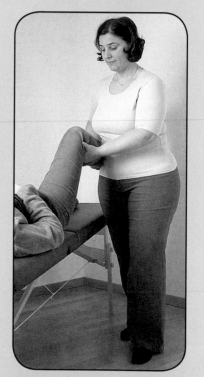

Figure 8.18

continued

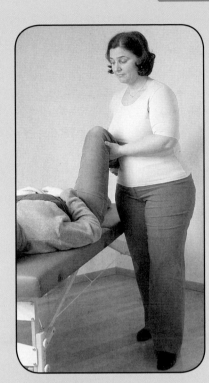

Figure 8.19

Partner feedback

How did these lifting techniques affect the quality of your movements?

_____

_____

How secure did your partner feel with these techniques?

_____

_____

Discuss the advantages of lifting, using the techniques in this lesson.

_____

_____

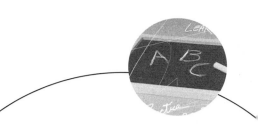

Client education tip 8.3

For many reasons, people hesitate to ask for help. However, encouraging your clients to ask for assistance in situations where they cannot lift and /or carry a heavy object by themselves can help prevent a serious accident from occurring. Assure them that asking for assistance is far less painful than enduring an injury that was preventable.

Ask for help

Before you start to lift any amount of weight, check in with yourself to make sure you feel comfortable lifting it. If you are uncomfortable for any reason, ask for help. For example, ask your client to move closer to you and/or help with the initiation of the lifting. If needed, you can also ask for help with holding and moving. Never feel embarrassed or inadequate when asking for assistance. Your first priority is your body's comfort and safety, and in keeping with this rule, you are a positive role model for your clients, as well.

When utilizing sheets and/or supports, such as bolsters, blocks or rollers, do not hesitate to ask your client to help you. Positioning sheets and supports while lifting can be challenging. As long as they are able, your clients can help lift themselves.

Remember, an important part of healthy body mechanics is knowing when to ask for help!

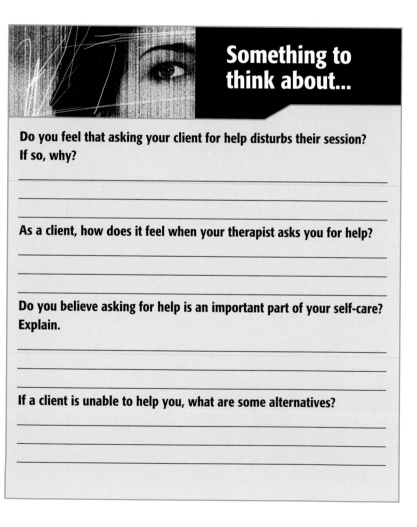

Something to think about...

Do you feel that asking your client for help disturbs their session? If so, why?

_____

_____

As a client, how does it feel when your therapist asks you for help?

_____

_____

Do you believe asking for help is an important part of your self-care? Explain.

_____

_____

If a client is unable to help you, what are some alternatives?

_____

_____

_____

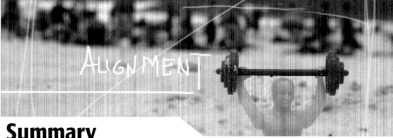

Summary

In this chapter, you have learned and experienced the importance of getting close and facing weight when lifting. You have also learned how to use the power of your legs and how to reduce stress in your upper body by lifting, holding and moving weight, using the support of your lower body. Here is a review of the concepts discussed in this chapter:

When lifting, **get** as **close** to the weight as possible, without leaning on your table for support. Getting as close as possible, no matter the amount of weight, is one of the simplest and smartest rules of proper lifting.

Face the weight to keep your body in proper alignment, eliminate rotation and decrease your strain and effort. Keep your feet, pelvis and upper body directed toward the weight to insure you are facing it without rotation.

Lift with your legs to allow your back to remain vertical and reduce excessive muscular effort in your shoulders, arms and hands. Your upper body facilitates the lifting, while the strong muscles of your legs do the hard work!

Life after lifting means that once you have lifted weight, you will probably want to move. If so, there are two good choices, both of which keep your back safe from injury:

The first choice is to remain in your original lifting position. From this position you can move while facing the weight, moving the client's leg in the direction of the head or foot of the table. Your feet should be in a parallel stance and your legs in good alignment. When you need to make a large movement, take side-steps in either direction.

The second choice is to reposition yourself while holding the weight. This means *after* you have lifted the leg, reposition yourself to fully face the intended direction of movement, e.g., the head of the table. Your feet should be in a one-foot forward stance and your legs in a good alignment. If you need to make a large movement, take steps forward or back.

Ask for help if you are uncomfortable, for any reason, with lifting any amount of weight.

Now that you've read this chapter...

When working, how aware are you of your lifting habits?
- almost always
- sometimes
- not very often
- other_____

When lifting, what parts of your body are you now most aware of?
- neck and shoulders
- arms and hands
- pelvis and legs
- other_____

When lifting, what parts of your body are you still not aware of?
- head and neck
- shoulders and upper back
- pelvis and legs
- other_____

Describe 5 concepts that make lifting more dynamic.
1. _____
2. _____
3. _____
4. _____
5. _____

Describe an aspect of lifting that feels easy and comfortable.
_____
_____

Describe an aspect of lifting that you do not feel comfortable with yet.
_____
_____

Now how confident are you lifting?
- completely
- mostly
- a little
- not at all

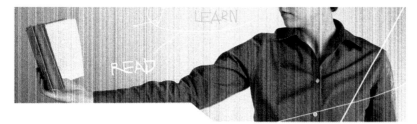

References

1. Niemiec, Nicole. *Lifting Techniques You Should Follow to Avoid Injuries to Your Back.* www.britain.tv/health. 27 May 2003.

2. Winters, Margaret C. *Protective Body Mechanics in Daily Life and in Nursing.* Philadelphia: W. B. Saunders, 1952.

3. *Lifting Techniques.* www.back.com. 2003. 26 May 2003.

4. *Safe Lifting Procedures.* City and County of Honolulu. Department of Human Resources. Division of Industrial Safety and Workers' Compensation.

5. *American Journal of Public Health.* 1994, Vol. 84, No. 11.

9 *Pushing and Pulling*

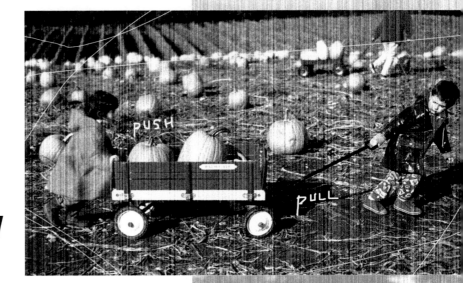

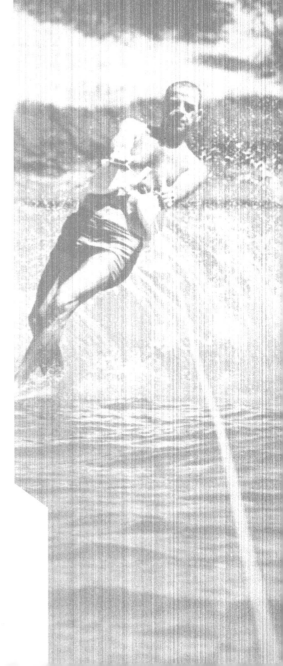

Introduction

Pushing and pulling, used together or separately, are major functions of all manual therapies. Whether manipulating bone, soft tissue or energy, the movements of pushing and pulling are inherent to the process. Sometimes the actions of pushing and pulling are obvious, as in chiropractic adjustments, massage therapy strokes and physical therapy manipulations. With other modalities, such as cranial-sacral work, myofascial release and energy work, pushing and pulling are used in subtler, but still very critical ways.

In this chapter you will learn to maintain self-support, generate strength with your lower body, utilize the concept of counterbalance, and align your shoulders, arms and hands. Together, these concepts will assist you to push and pull dynamically and effectively.

The concepts learned in Chapters 5 and 7 will be discussed in this chapter. If needed, go back and review these chapters before continuing on.

Before you read this chapter…

How often do you push and pull on a daily basis?

- *almost always*
- *sometimes*
- *not very often*
- *other*_____

What parts of your body are you most aware of when pushing and pulling?

- *head and neck*
- *shoulders and upper back*
- *pelvis and legs*
- *other*_____

What parts of your body are you least aware of when pushing and pulling?

- *head and neck*
- *shoulders and upper back*
- *pelvis and legs*
- *other*_____

Describe 5 pushing and pulling activities that you do on a regular basis.

(e.g., vacuuming, lawn mowing, opening doors…)

1. _____
2. _____
3. _____
4. _____
5. _____

Describe an everyday activity involving pushing and/or pulling that you do with ease and comfort.

_____
_____

Describe an everyday activity involving pushing and/or pulling that you do with difficulty or discomfort.

_____
_____

How comfortable are you pushing and/or pulling on an everyday basis?

- *always*
- *mostly*
- *sometimes*
- *very seldom*

Self-supported pushing

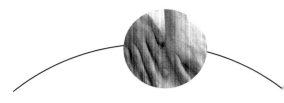

A crucial component in developing a healthy self-care strategy is maintaining a sense of self- support throughout your treatments. When this element is present, your body mechanics are sound, increasing the sensitivity and effectiveness of your touch. Therefore, when pushing, rely on *your* body for stability and support, not on your client's. Self-supported pushing means bending from your hip joints and knees, counterbalancing your pelvis and upper body, distributing your weight and using your feet in full contact with the floor. In this instance, your lower body is in the position for powerful pushing while your upper body is free to move, allowing your arms and hands to push effectively.[1] (9.1) Using body weight to gain strength is appropriate, using your client's body for support and stability is not.

Practice tip 9.1

When you find that you are relying on your client's body for support, bring your attention to your feet. Notice if they are in full contact with the floor and if you are utilizing your "tripods." (See Ch. 5, page 111.) If not, readjust your stance, bring your feet in contact with the floor and use the concepts of Partner practice 9.1. Supporting yourself with your feet prevents stress on your hands and decreases the muscular effort in your upper body, such as your back and shoulders.

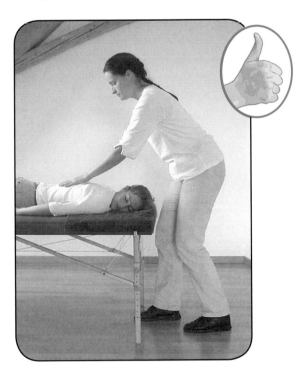

Figure 9.1

If, at any point during your pushing you begin to lean into your client's body, in such a way that you lose your stability, you compromise your body mechanics. (9.2) An easy way to check this, is to take your hands away from your client's body while pushing, and notice if you begin to fall forward. If so, you have lost your self-support. When this happens, the only function your hands can manage is that of supporting you by way of your client's body, eliminating the chance to perform the specific pushing techniques required. Furthermore, the rest of your body must work hard to compensate for your lack of balance

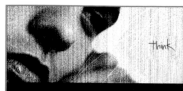

Something to think about...

What kind of objects do you push during a normal day? (e.g., a drawer, door, cart...)

_____

_____

When you push, what parts of your body do you sense yourself using?

_____

_____

When working, how often do you use pushing techniques?

_____

_____

Do you feel that you maintain your sense of self-support when pushing? If not, explain.

_____

_____

_____

_____

_____

_____

and self-support. The quality of your treatment is compromised when your hands do not have the control needed for sensitive touch.

When you maintain your self-support while pushing, you push with effectiveness and, at the same time, remain in control. The following *Partner practice* lesson will give you the opportunity to experience this concept.

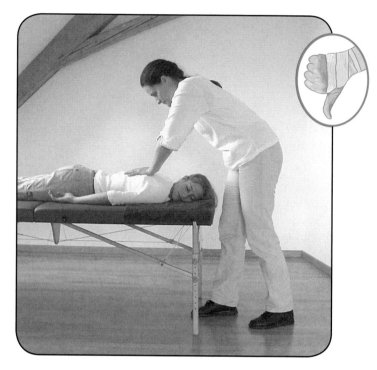

Figure 9.2

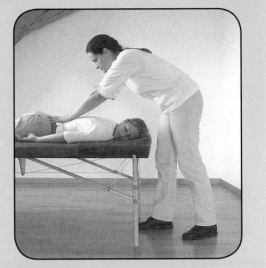

Self-supported pushing

Ask your partner to lie supine on your table. Stand in a way that requires you to use your partner's body for your support. Slowly begin to push your hands down your partner's back. When you reach the lower back, stop and remain in this position for a few minutes. (9.3)

Sense how your hands and wrist joints respond when pushing in this way.
How much control and sensitivity do you have in your hands right now?
How comfortable do your hands and wrist joints feel?
Where in your hands do you feel most of the stress when pushing in this way?
What would happen if you were to quickly remove your hands from your partner's back?

Figure 9.3

Notice the effort in your neck, back and shoulders.
Is there an increase of muscular effort in your neck?
Is there an increase of effort in your back?
Is there an increase of effort in your shoulders?

Sense the amount of control and balance that you have in your legs and feet.
Are your feet able to maintain contact with the ground?
Do you sense an increase of effort in your legs?
Do you feel balanced and in control?

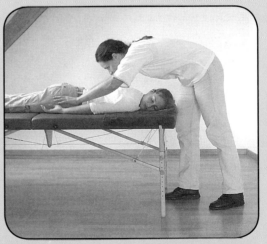

Notice if you are able to breathe comfortably.
How is your breathing affected when pushing this way?

Now quickly remove your hands from your partner's back. (9.4)
What happens to your balance?
Do you begin to fall into your partner's body?

Now replace your hands on your partner's lower back and

Figure 9.4

continued

begin to pull your hands up his or her back. (9.5)

Sense the effort it takes to pull away from your pushing.
Is the effort centered in your neck and shoulders?
Is the effort centered in your back?
Do you sense the effort in your hands and wrist joints?

Rest.

Stand vertically aligned and use the tripods of your feet.
Begin to bend from your hip joints, knees and ankles, and
counterbalance your pelvis and upper body. Be sure to keep
your feet in full contact with the floor. Now, slowly push your
hands down your partner's back. When you reach the lower
back, stop and remain in this position for a few minutes. (9.6)

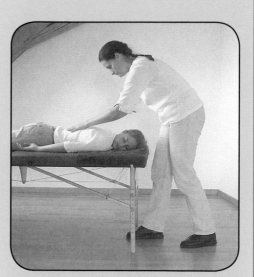

Figure 9.5

Sense the amount of sensitivity and control you have in
your hands.
How much control and sensitivity do you have in your hands
right now?
How comfortable do your hands and wrist joints feel?
Do you sense stress in your hands when pushing in this way?
What would happen if you were to quickly remove your hands
from your partner's back?

Notice the response in your neck, back and shoulders.
Is there a decrease of muscular effort in your neck?
Is there a decrease of effort in your back?
Is there a decrease of effort in your shoulders?

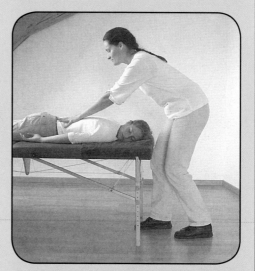

Figure 9.6

Sense the amount of control and balance you have in your
legs and feet.
Are your feet able to maintain contact with the ground?
Do you sense a decrease of effort in your legs?
Do you feel balanced and in control?

Notice if you are able to breathe comfortably.
Can you breathe comfortably?

Now quickly remove your hands from your partner's back. (9.7)
What happens to your balance?
Do you maintain your balance over your partner's body?
Do you feel self-supported?

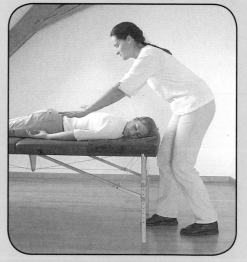

Figure 9.7

continued

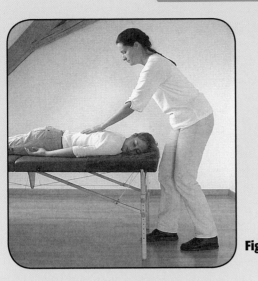

Figure 9.8

Now replace your hands on your partner's lower back and begin to pull your hands up his or her back. **(9.8)**

Sense the response of your body when pulling away.
Is there less effort centered in your hands and wrist joints?
Is there less effort in your neck, shoulders and back?
Are your legs and feet able to facilitate the pulling?
Do you feel self-supported?

Rest.

By pushing in a self-supportive manner you become self-reliant, using your own body to push with effectiveness, confidence, and increasing your overall control and sensitivity.

Partner feedback
What did your partner feel when using his or her body for your support?

_____

_____

How much control and sensitivity could he or she sense in your hands when using his/her body for your support?

_____

_____

What qualities changed when you became self-supported?

_____

_____

_____

_____

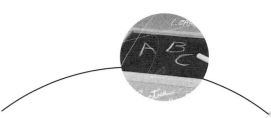

Client education tip 9.1

Household activities requiring pushing, such as vacuuming and lawn mowing, can be difficult when the strength of the upper body is primarily used for power. Explain the concept of using the lower body for strength to those clients who are experiencing difficulties with pushing activities. You can even lead them through the first part of Partner practice 9.2 . Who knows, it may just make household tasks more pleasurable!

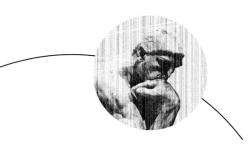

The pushing power of your lower body

When pushing, sometimes you wil require a lot of power, but sometimes not. How do you acquire the necessary strength and, at the same time, allow your upper body to remain stress-free? The answer lies in the counterbalance and strength of your lower body. As you have learned, counterbalancing your pelvis and upper body increases stability. You have also learned that your hip joints are the strongest and most stable joints, that your legs, when aligned, are powerful tools, and that your feet support your weight. Together, all of these concepts play an important role when it comes to safe, yet powerful pushing.

When executing pushing techniques, manual therapists often use the power of the upper body to generate the required strength. This style of pushing forces the upper back, shoulders, arms and hands to produce an enormous amount of power, compromising the integrity of the muscles and joints involved. (9.9)

Bending from your hip joints, knees and ankles and counterbalancing with proper leg alignment, puts you in the optimal position for powerful pushing. This posture allows you to press your feet into the floor as you push your upper body forward, maintain your self-support and increase your power and strength tenfold. This style of pushing relies on the strength of your lower body, relieving your hands of forceful work and giving you a sense of overall control. (9.10)

The following *Partner practice* lesson illustrates this concept.

Consider this

Every event in track and field utilizes the concept of pressing the feet to push the body forward. Relay races, hurdling, steeplechase, high jump, pole vault, long jump, triple jump, shot put, discus throw, hammer throw and javelin throw, all require the athlete to use his lower body in a powerful and explosive way to propel and push his upper body forward.

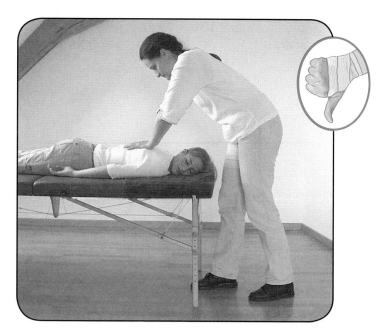

Figure 9.9

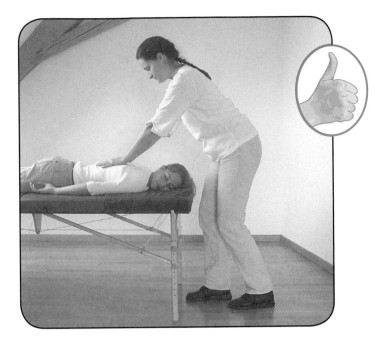

Figure 9.10

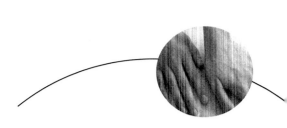

Practice tip 9.2

When you sense that your upper body begins to fatigue, especially your shoulders, notice if you are using your lower body to generate power. If not, relax your hands, arms and shoulders, and let your lower body provide the power you need. This will decrease the stress on your upper body. If your upper body is primarily used to generate power, the muscles and joints of your shoulders, arms and hands will quickly fatigue and become strained. Use the larger muscles and joints of your lower body for power and save the smaller muscles and joints of your upper body from injury.

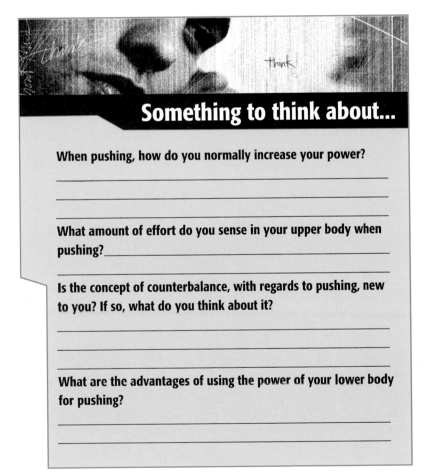

Something to think about...

When pushing, how do you normally increase your power?

_____
_____
_____

What amount of effort do you sense in your upper body when pushing? _____
_____

Is the concept of counterbalance, with regards to pushing, new to you? If so, what do you think about it?

_____
_____
_____

What are the advantages of using the power of your lower body for pushing?

_____
_____

Powerful pushing

Stand by a wall and lean all of your weight onto it. Begin to push on the wall, as if you would like to push it over. (9.11)

Notice how you use your body to push the wall.
What parts of your body do you use to push with?
Are you using your shoulder, arms and hands to push it over?
Are your feet pressing into the ground as you push?
How much strength can you generate pushing in this manner?

Be careful with this next action.
Now quickly take your hands away from the wall.

Did you lose your balance and fall into the wall?

Rest.

Stand again by the wall, in a self-supported manner, with your legs and feet aligned, counterbalancing your pelvis and upper body. Begin again to push into the wall, as if to push it over. (9.12)

Tip Press your feet into the floor as you push your hands on the wall.

Notice how your body responds to pushing in this manner.
How much stronger is your pushing compared to before?
Where is most of your strength coming from?
Do you sense an increase of power when pressing your feet into the floor?

Quickly take your hands away from the wall.

Did you lose your balance this time?

Tip Counterbalancing your pelvis and upper body will help you maintain your self-support, keeping you from falling into the wall.

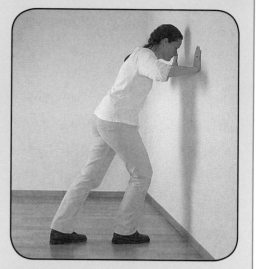

Figure 9.11

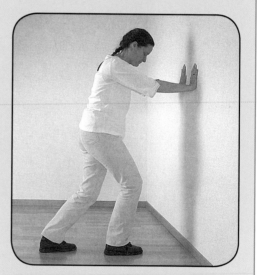

Figure 9.12

continued

Rest.

Now ask your partner to lie prone on your table and stand at the head of the table. Begin to push your hands into your partner's back, leaning all of your weight to generate your power. Do not move your hands down the back just yet. (9.13)

Notice how your body responds to this style of pushing.
Where is the focus of your pushing?
How does this style affect your hands and wrist joints?
Do you feel that you have control and balance?
What would happen if you were to quickly take your hands away?

Begin to push your hands down your partner's back. Slowly increase the power of your pushing by leaning more of your weight onto your partner's body. (Check in with your partner to make sure you are not hurting them.)

Notice again your body's response to your pushing.
How much effort is required to increase the power to push in this manner?
How is the quality of your touch affected?
Do you sense increased effort in your shoulders, arms and hands?
What would happen if you were to quickly take your hands away from your partner's back?

Rest.

Now stand in a self-supported manner. Bend from your hip joints, knees and ankles, and counterbalance your pelvis and upper body. Begin to press your feet into the floor as you slowly begin to push into your partner's back. Do not move down the back, just push into the back and then release the pressure. Practice this several times. (9.14)

Notice how your body responds to this style of pushing.
Where is the focus of your pushing?
Is the focus of your pushing now in your feet and legs?
Do you feel that you have control and balance?
What would happen if you were to quickly take your hands away?

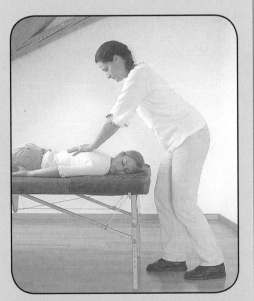

Figure 9.13

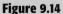

Figure 9.14

continued

Begin to move your hands down your partner's back. Remain self-supported and use the pressing of your feet to lengthen your upper body as you push your hands down your partner's back. (9.15)

Rest.

Stand as before, and again push your hands into your partner's back. Begin to slowly increase the power of your push by pressing your feet into the floor a little more.

Now begin to push your hands down your partner's back. Continue to press your feet, using your lower body to generate strength. As you move your hands down the back, lengthen your body, maintaining your balance and control. Focus on incorporating the movement of your entire body into your pushing.

Tip Do not move your hands so far down the back that you lose your balance and control. Stop *before* you compromise your balance.

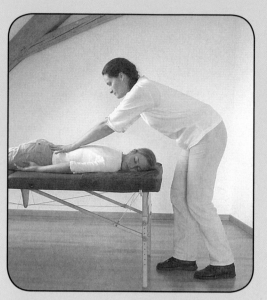

Figure 9.15

Notice your body's response to generating power in this manner.
How much effort is required from your hands to increase power in this manner?
Has the sensitivity of your touch improved?
Do you sense the advantages of pressing your feet into the floor to generate the power to push?
Do you have a sense of control and self-support?

Rest.

Generate the required power to push by pressing your feet into the floor. This concept utilizes the strength of your lower body while allowing your upper body to execute your therapy with ease and proficiency.

Partner feedback
How was the quality of your touch affected when you were leaning all of your weight onto your partner's body?

_____

_____

How was the quality and the strength of your pushing influenced when you were maintaining your balance and pressing your feet into the floor?

_____

_____

Which style of pushing felt most effective to you and your partner?

_____

_____

Pushing with alignment

Though all of the concepts mentioned so far are important, if you do not maintain your skeletal alignment when pushing, you may still lack the effectiveness and comfort you desire.

When pushing and using the power of your lower body, you are generating and transmitting force from your feet up to your hands. If the force you generate travels up through a well-aligned skeleton, you create a strong and healthy pathway. (9.16) However, if the force you create travels through a misaligned skeleton, stress will accumulate in the areas of misalignment and your body mechanics will be compromised. (9.17)

Take a few minutes to experience the following *Self-observation* lesson. It will help you understand this concept.

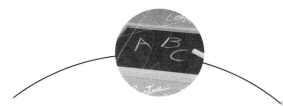

Client education tip 9.2

If you have a client who is experiencing pain in a joint, such as the elbow, notice his or her skeletal alignment. Ask what kind of activity exacerbates the pain and ask him/her to show you how he/she move during the activity. For instance, if typing on the computer causes pain in the elbows, notice if the elbows are held out to the side instead of in alignment with the shoulders and wrist joints. Bringing attention to alignment can often help relieve joint pain.

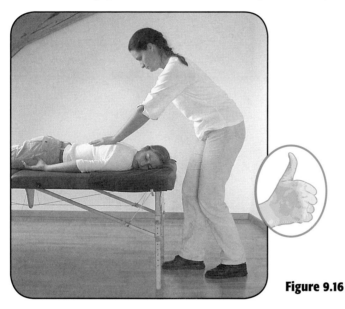

Figure 9.16

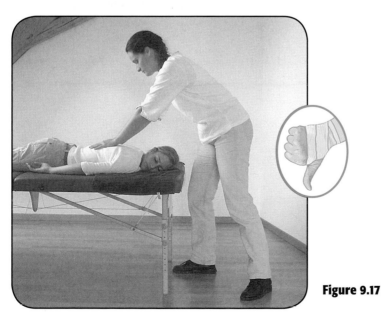

Figure 9.17

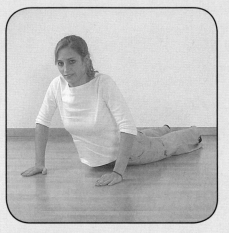

Pushing with skeletal alignment

Lie on the floor, on your stomach. Place your hands in a "push up" position, shoulder width apart. Slowly begin to push your upper body away from the floor by pressing your hands into the floor. (9.19)

Tip Make sure your hands are comfortably aligned with your elbows and your elbows with your shoulders. In this position you create a "bridge" of support.

Do you sense the strength of your skeletal alignment as you push yourself away from the floor?
How much muscular effort is needed?

Now move your hands outside the width of your shoulders. (9.20)

Does this position make the pushing easier or harder?
How much muscular effort is needed?
Where do you feel the effort in your body?

Now move your hands inside the width of your shoulders. (9.21)

Does this make the pushing easier or harder?
How much muscular effort is needed?
Where do you feel the effort in your body?

Rest.

Bring your hands back underneath your shoulders and push yourself up again.

Notice the strength and support you have when pushing with an aligned skeleton.
Has your muscular effort decreased?

Pushing yourself away from the floor can help you sense the importance of skeletal alignment. When using manual pushing techniques, you can use the same principle. Use proper alignment to decrease muscular effort and increase your strength by utilizing your skeleton.

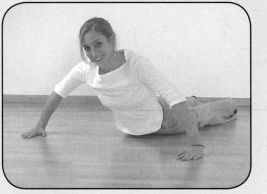

Figure 9.19

Figure 9.20

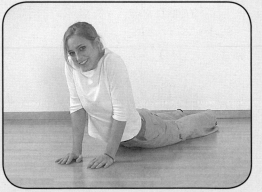

Figure 9.21

continued

Self-feedback

How was your strength affected when your hands were outside shoulders' width?

_____

_____

_____

How was your strength affected when your hands were inside shoulders' width?

_____

_____

_____

What qualities of strength did you sense when your shoulders, elbows and hands were aligned?

_____

_____

_____

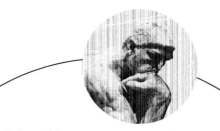

Consider this

At about 6 months of age, a baby will intuitively push her upper body up with her hands when lying on her stomach. She positions herself in such a way that she uses the strength of her aligned skeleton to do the pushing, creating a "bridge" of support with her hands, arms and chest. [2] *(9.18)*

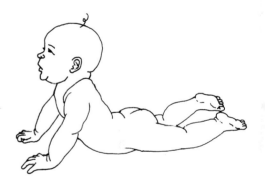

Figure 9.18

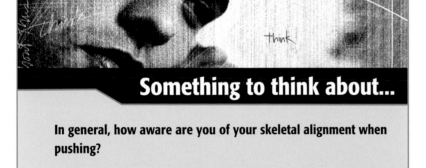

Something to think about...

In general, how aware are you of your skeletal alignment when pushing?

_____

_____

When pushing, have you ever sensed your skeleton to be misaligned? Explain. _____

_____

_____

How can an aligned skeleton increase the effectiveness of your pushing?

_____

_____

_____

Self-supported pulling

Self-support is as important while pulling as it is while pushing. Whether pulling subtly with your fingers or pulling forcefully with your hands, you must pull using the support of your body, not your client's, to maintain effective body mechanics and quality of touch. Self-supported pulling means counterbalancing your pelvis and upper body, using the power of your lower body to pull and remaining in full control of your balance. (9.22)

The tendency when pulling is to lean back and suspend all of the body's weight through the hands, arms and shoulders. An example of this kind of pulling is the game of "tug-of-war" where two teams of people pull opposite ends of a rope. The team who pulls the other team across the middle line wins. Due to a non-supportive style of pulling, if either team lets go of the rope, the other team falls quickly backward to the ground. This style of pulling is also seen in manual therapy. It is common to see a therapist pull (traction), for example a leg, by leaning the body's weight back, relying on the client's leg for balance. (9.23) If the therapist were to release her hands quickly, or if the leg slipped from her hands, she would fall backward.

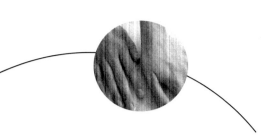

Practice tip 9.3

The next time you are performing a pulling type of technique, become aware of your hands. Check in and sense the amount of effort you are using. If you find that you are gripping tightly, try using more of your lower body and let your hands relax. Use the strength of your lower body and allow your hands to pull with sensitivity.

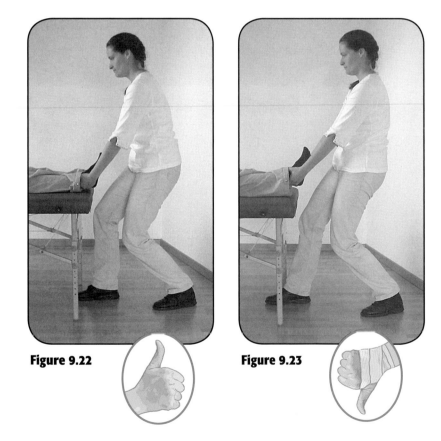

Figure 9.22 **Figure 9.23**

As with pushing, if, at any point during pulling, you begin to use your body's weight in such a way that you lose your sense of self-support, you compromise your body mechanics. A way to check this is to release your hands from your client and notice if you begin to fall backward.

Self-supported pulling allows you to pull effectively, while remaining in full control of your balance. The following *Partner practice* lesson gives you the opportunity to experience this concept.

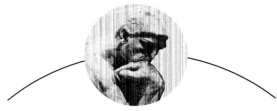

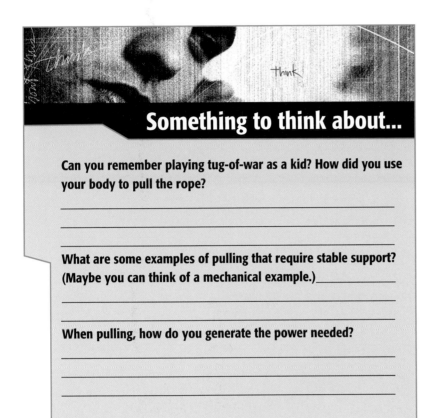

Something to think about...

Can you remember playing tug-of-war as a kid? How did you use your body to pull the rope?

_____

_____

_____

What are some examples of pulling that require stable support? (Maybe you can think of a mechanical example.)_____

_____

_____

When pulling, how do you generate the power needed?

_____

_____

_____

Consider this

The function of pulling starts at a very early age. Shortly after birth, a baby will begin to grasp and pull at his mother's breast while feeding. At the age of about 6 months, a baby will lie on his back and pull his feet toward his mouth.[3]

Self-supported pulling

Stand at the head of your table. Pull your table with your hands, leaning back with your body weight. **(9.24)** *(Ask your partner to hold the other end of the table so it remains in place.)*

Notice how your body weight is suspended from your table.
What would happen if you were to suddenly let go of your table?

Notice how your body responds to this style of pulling.
Do you sense muscular effort in your shoulders, arms and hands?
Do you feel strain in your hands and wrist joints?
Do you sense effort in your upper back and neck?
Do you sense effort in your legs and feet?

Notice how this kind of pulling affects your breathing.
Is your breathing restricted in any way?

Rest.

Now stand in a self-supported manner. Bend from your hip joints, knees and ankles, and counterbalance your pelvis and upper body. Slowly begin to pull on your table again. **(9.25)** *(Ask you partner to hold the other end.)*

Notice how you are now able to counterbalance the weight of your body, instead of suspending it from the table, as before.
What would happen if you were to suddenly let go of your table now?

Notice how your body responds to this style of pulling.
Has the control and sensitivity increased in your hands?
Do you feel less strain on your hand and wrist joints?
Can you let your hands pull without overly gripping your table?
Has the effort in your shoulders and back decreased?
Has the effort in your legs and feet decreased?

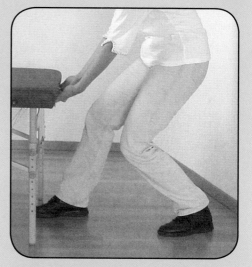

Figure 9.24

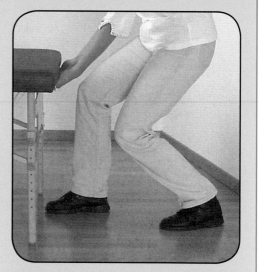

Figure 9.25

continued

Rest.

Ask your partner to lie supine on your table. Slowly begin to pull your partner's leg by leaning back, using his/her leg for your support. (9.26)

Notice how your lack of self-support influences your quality of touch.
Do you have a sense of control and sensitivity in your hands?
Do you feel effort in your hands?

Notice your body's response to this style of pulling.
Do you sense effort in your shoulders?
Has the effort in your back and legs increased?
Are your feet in contact with the ground?
What would happen if you were to suddenly let go of your partner's leg?

Rest.

Now stand in a self-supported manner. Bend from your hip joints, knees and ankles, and counterbalance your pelvis and upper body. Slowly begin to pull your partner's leg. (9.27)

Notice how your self-support increases your quality of touch.
Do you feel less strain on your hands and wrists?
Can you let your hands pull without overly gripping your table?

Notice your body's response to this style of pulling.
Has the effort in your shoulders decreased?
Has the effort in your back and legs decreased?
Are your feet able to remain in contact with the ground?
If you were to let go, could you maintain your sense of self-support?

Rest.

A self-supportive style of pulling is the most effective way to pull and maintain balance. Pulling in this manner assures, you and your client, that the specific pulling techniques required are being executed with the utmost care and safety.

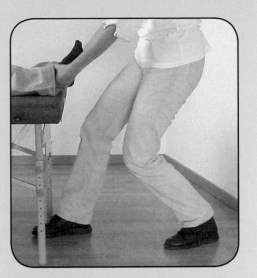

Figure 9.26

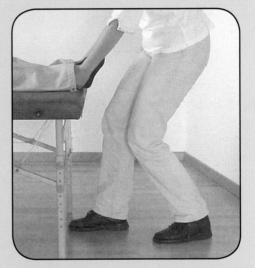

Figure 9.27

continued

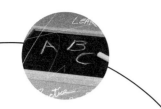

Client education tip 9.3

If you work with athletes, share the concept of pressing down and pulling back. Though they might know it unconsciously, bringing their attention to this concept can help make their sport more dynamic. When more of the body is consciously integrated into an activity, less stress is likely to accumulate in specific areas.

Partner feedback

How was the quality of your touch affected when you suspended your weight from your partner's leg?

_____

_____

How was your touch influenced when you maintained your balance with your own body?

_____

_____

Which style of pulling felt the safest and most effective to you and your partner? Explain.

_____

_____

_____

_____

Something to think about...

Have you ever rowed a boat? Think about how you propelled the boat through the water. What movements did your legs and arms make simultaneously?

_____

_____

_____

If you have never rowed, during what other kinds of activities have you experienced the pressing of your feet and the pulling of your upper body?_____

_____

Is this concept of pulling new to you? If so, what do you think of it? _____

_____

_____

_____

_____

Pressing down and pulling back

Have you ever watched the movement of a skilled rower? As he pulls back on the oars with his hands, he presses his feet into the boat. This simultaneous pressing and pulling generates the power needed to move the boat through the water at an impressive speed.[4] You can use this same kind of movement to generate power when pulling as well.

When sitting, the rowing example translates easily into practice, but when standing, you must add the component of counterbalance to the process. Counterbalancing helps you maintain your balance while using your lower body to generate power. Using counterbalance, you can effectively press your feet into the ground as you pull back with your hands. Pulling in this fashion does not isolate the pulling action in one area, for example, your hands, but rather uses your entire body to pull with power and stability.

The following *Partner practice* is a fun way to experience this concept.

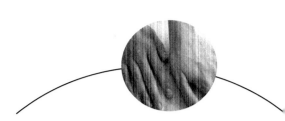

Practice tip 9.4

It is said that with every pushing action, there is a pulling action that follows. Considering this, pulling is an inherent part of your work. During your next session, become aware of how often you intentionally pull and how often you pull due to a pushing action. Becoming aware of this can help clarify the need for sound 'pulling' body mechanics.

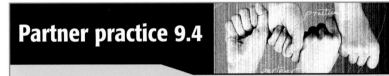

Partner practice 9.4

Pulling with power

Preparation You will need a piece of rope to play a game of tug-of-war.

Stand and hold the end of a piece of rope - your partner holds the other end. On the count of three, ask your partner to begin pulling the rope, while you pull as well. Play a friendly game of tug-of-war with each other.

Notice how you use your body to pull the rope.
How are you generating your power?
Does your power come from your upper body?
Does your power come from your legs and feet?
What would happen if your partner were to let go of the rope?

Rest for a moment.

Stand in a self-supported manner, counterbalancing your pelvis and upper body. Begin to play again. As you begin to pull the rope, press your feet into the ground, maintaining your self-support. To increase your strength, increase the pressing of your feet into the ground. If needed, take steps backward. **(9.28)**

Notice how your body responds to this style of pulling.

How are you now generating your power?

Does your power come from your upper, lower or entire body?

Has your strength increased?

What would happen if you or your partner were to let go of the rope?

Rest.

Now ask your partner to lie supine on your table. Slowly begin to pull her/his leg while maintaining your self-support and pressing your feet into the floor. (9.29)

Now stop pulling in this manner and begin to pull by suspending your weight from the leg.

Notice the difference between the two styles of pulling.

Which one feels more effective?

Stop again and begin pulling, as before, maintaining your support and pressing your feet into the floor. Continue to pull for a few moments and then stop. Repeat this a few times.

Tip If you find that you are primarily pulling using the strength of your hands and wrists, try to reduce the amount of effort you are using in your hands. If your lower body is supporting you, your hands can facilitate the pulling without overly gripping.

Rest.

Pull your partner's leg again as before. Slowly begin to increase the strength of pulling by increasing the pressing of your feet into the ground. While pressing, you may feel as if you would like to take a step back. This is fine, just make sure you maintain your self-support. (9.30)

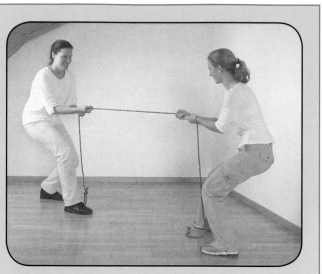

Figure 9.28

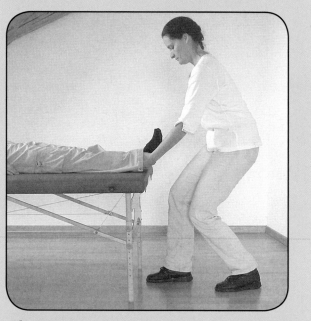

Figure 9.29

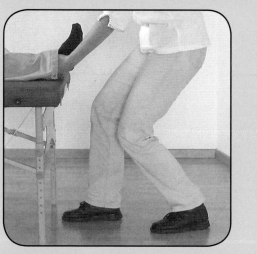

Figure 9.30

continued

Notice how pressing your feet affects your strength.
How much effort is needed to increase your strength?
Are you able to let your entire body facilitate the pulling without stressing your hands?

Rest.

Once again, pull your partner's leg. Slowly begin to increase the amount of pull, as before, and now decrease the amount of pull by pressing less into the floor. Even though you are pressing less with your feet and decreasing your pull, continue to remain self-supported. Practice increasing and decreasing your pulling strength several times, fine tuning your skill.

Notice the amount of control you have.
Are you easily able to increase and decrease the strength of your pulling?

Rest.

Pulling using counterbalance while pressing with your feet, increases your strength without compromising your balance, giving you the control needed to make obvious and subtle changes. Your entire body is used dynamically instead of focusing all the effort in your hands.

Partner feedback
What were the differences between the two styles of pulling?

_____
_____
_____

How did the two styles of pulling affect the quality of your touch?

_____
_____
_____

How did the two styles of pulling affect the quality of your control?

_____
_____
_____

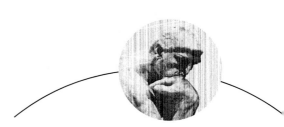

Consider this

To counterbalance the weight of her rig, a windsurfer must balance her pelvis and upper body by pressing down on the board with her feet and pulling back on the mast with her hands. This allows her to maintain balance while sailing. Without the element of counterbalance she would spend most of her time in the water, instead of on her board! [5]

Now that you've read this chapter...

When working, how aware are you now of your pushing and pulling habits?
- *almost always*
- *sometimes*
- *not very often*
- *other_____*

When pushing and pulling, what parts of your body are you now most aware of?
- *neck and shoulders*
- *arms and hands*
- *pelvis and legs*
- *other_____*

When pushing and pulling, what parts of your body are you still not aware of?
- *neck and shoulders*
- *arms and hands*
- *pelvis and legs*
- *other_____*

Describe 5 concepts that make your pushing and pulling more dynamic.

1. _____
2. _____
3. _____
4. _____
5. _____

Describe an aspect of pushing or pulling that is easy and comfortable.

_____

_____

Describe an aspect of pushing or pulling that is not yet easy and comfortable.

_____

_____

How comfortable are you now pushing and pulling?
- *completely*
- *mostly*
- *a little bit*
- *not very*

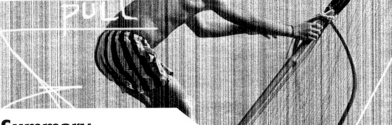

Summary

In this chapter, you have learned how to maintain self-support, generate strength with your lower body, utilize the concept of counterbalance and align your shoulders, arms and hands. Together, these concepts have helped you push and pull dynamically and effectively. Here is a review of the concepts learned in this chapter:

Self-supported pushing means bending from your hip joints and knees, counterbalancing your pelvis and upper body, distributing your weight and using your feet in full contact with the floor. In this instance, your lower body is in the position for powerful pushing while your upper body is free to move, allowing your arms and hands to push effectively.

The pushing power of your lower body is utilized when you counterbalance, bend from your hip joints, and *press* your feet into the floor as you *push* your upper body forward. This helps you maintain your self-support and increases your power and strength tenfold.

When you push with proper **skeletal alignment**, the force you create travels up through a strong and powerful pathway.

Self-supported pulling means counterbalancing your pelvis and upper body, using the power of your lower body to pull and remaining in full control of your balance.

When **pressing down and pulling back**, you do not isolate the pulling action in one area, for example, your hands, but rather use your entire body to pull with power and stability.

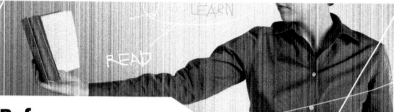

References

1. Haller, Jeff. *Feldenkrais Professional Training Program.* Maui, Hawaii, 1994.

2. *Die Entwicklung im 1. Lebensjahr.* www.home.wtal.de/uerhage/ babyentwicklung. 3 April 2000.

3. Begley, Sharon. *The Nature of Nurturing. Newsweek Special Magazine.* March 2000.

4. Wetzler, Brad. *The Push/ Pull.* www.outsidemag.com. July 1997: Summer Special: The Push and Pull.

5. *Wind Surfing Techniques.* www.windsurfing.com. June 2003.

10 Applying Pressure

LIGHT PRESSURE

Introduction

No matter what kind of manual therapy you practice, the one function which remains constant is the application of pressure. Whether pressing lightly with your fingertips or applying deep pressure with your hands, forearms or elbows, whether pushing or pulling you are, to some degree, constantly applying pressure.

Applying pressure is a form of pushing, and although you have learned how to push effectively, it is still prudent to focus on familiar topics such as applying pressure by using your body weight, effective alignment, getting close to your work, and how breathing can help your body stay dynamic when applying sustained pressure. Together these concepts will increase your effectiveness and keep your body mechanics dynamic.

If needed, review Chapter 9 before continuing on.

Before you read this chapter...

How often do you apply pressure to something on a regular basis?

- almost always
- sometimes
- not very often
- other_____

What parts of your body are you most aware of when applying pressure?

- head and neck
- shoulders and upper back
- pelvis and legs
- other_____

What parts of your body are you least aware of when applying pressure?

- head and neck
- shoulders and upper back
- pelvis and legs
- other_____

Describe 5 activities during which you apply pressure.

(e.g., waxing your car, brushing your teeth, cleaning windows, polishing furniture...)

1. _____
2. _____
3. _____
4. _____
5. _____

Describe an everyday activity in which you apply pressure with ease and comfort.

_____

_____

Describe an everyday activity in which you apply pressure with effort and discomfort.

_____

_____

How comfortable are you when applying pressure on a regular basis?

- always
- mostly
- sometimes
- seldom

Get close to apply pressure

In Chapter 8, you learned about the advantages of getting close when lifting. There are also advantages to getting close when working in general and when applying pressure, in particular.

Whenever possible, position yourself close to your area of focus. Rather than having to reach, causing unnecessary effort, working close to your client allows you better access to your focal point. (10.1) Though this is a somewhat obvious concept, many therapists find themselves working several inches away from their client, putting strain on the entire body, especially on the shoulders, arms and hands. (10.2) Working close to your client decreases your fatigue and greatly reduces your overall effort.

Working close is especially important when it comes to applying pressure. Because applying pressure often involves holding the same position for several seconds, you need to keep your body as relaxed as possible. If you are standing several inches away and, at the same time, holding sustained pressure, you are asking your body to work overtime. There is no need to stand far away. Make it easy on yourself and stand close enough so you do not need to strain to reach your client.

The following *Self-observation* lesson highlights this concept.

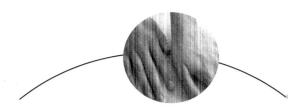

Practice tip 10.1

The next time you are out in public, notice the amount of space you need between yourself and others, for example, when talking to a stranger, with an acquaintance or a close friend. As a therapist, notice the amount of space between you and your client when talking. Does this space change depending on how well you know or like the client? Being aware of your social space can be very insightful.

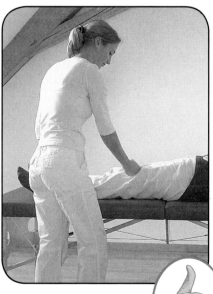

Figure 10.1

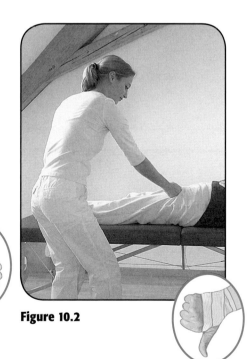

Figure 10.2

Getting close

Stand a few inches away from your table and, with both hands, apply some pressure to the edge of it. Stand far enough away so you need to reach out to apply the pressure. (10.3) (This might seem like an exaggeration but it will emphasize the point.)

Notice how your body responds to this distance.
Can you feel how much effort it takes to reach your table from where you are standing?
How stable and balanced are you?
How do the muscles of your arms and shoulders feel?
How are the muscles of your back and neck affected?
Where do you bend from, in order to reach your table?
Can you breathe easily from this position?
How effectively can you apply pressure?

Rest.

This time, stand close to your table, applying pressure to the edge. Stand in a self-supported manner, as previously learned. (10.4)

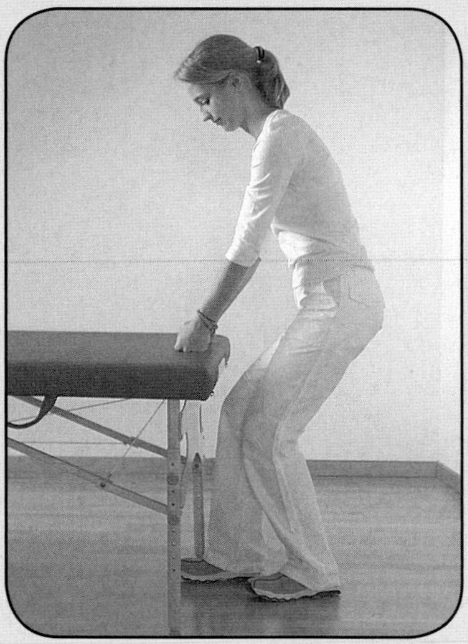

Notice how your body responds to this closer distance.
Can you now apply pressure using less effort?
Has your control and stability increased?
Are your arms and shoulders more relaxed now?
Is your back and neck more relaxed now?
Can you breathe easily from this position?
Can you apply pressure more effectively from this closer distance?

Rest.

Standing close when applying pressure increases your effectiveness and decreases the effort in your upper body.

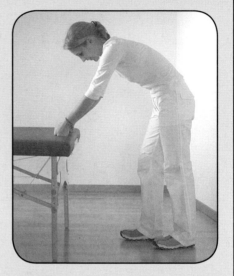

Figure 10.3

Figure 10.4

Self-feedback
What differences did you notice when applying pressure from a distance vs. applying pressure standing close? _____
_____

What are the disadvantages of applying pressure from a distance?
_____
_____

What are the advantages of standing close? _____
_____

Effective alignment

The advantages of skeletal alignment have been a theme throughout this book. We have explored the alignment of the entire skeleton and the alignment of the lower body. In the previous chapter we touched on the importance of finding the best shoulder, arm and hand alignment for pushing. Here, we will continue to focus on the upper body. This is not to imply that you should not pay attention to your complete skeletal alignment while applying pressure, but in this section we will emphasize the shoulders, arms and hands.

Effective alignment is a line of support which you create by stacking your bones in such a way that you sense and use the strength of your bones, as opposed to the effort of your muscles. Essentially, you sense skeletal support by transferring the force of pressure through bones, not muscles. When applying pressure, align your shoulder, elbow and wrist joint so that the strength of your bones do the work, not your muscles. In effect, you create a line of force with your skeleton to the contact point on the client's body. (10.5)

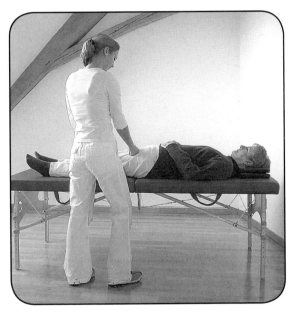

Figure 10.5

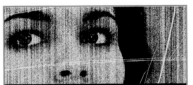

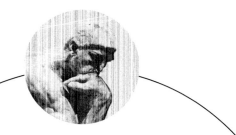

Applying pressure can stress the joints of the hand, arm and shoulder when poorly aligned. (10.6) Over time these joints become weak and unable to withstand such force. Keep your joints in alignment or "stacked" to ensure the integrity of your joints and allow the pressure to travel in a direct line. (10.7)

The following *Partner practice* gives you the opportunity to explore this concept.

Consider this

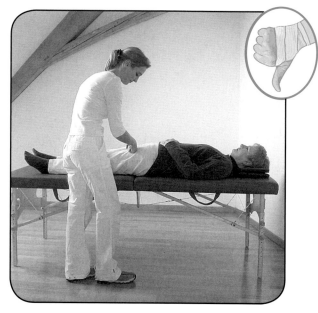

Figure 10.6

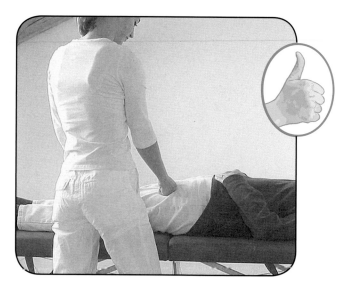

Figure 10.7

Partner practice 10.1

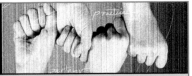

Finding effective alignment

Ask your partner to lie on his or her back. Stand by the side, in a self-supported manner. Apply pressure, with the top of your fist, to your partner's leg. Find an effective alignment which allows you to press comfortably and effectively from your standing position. (10.8)

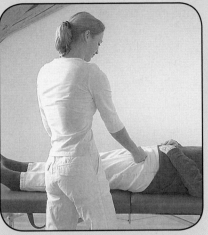

Figure 10.8

Tip Remember, the most effective alignment is one that keeps your joints "stacked". You should sense the strength of your alignment as you apply pressure.

Notice the strength of your alignment.
Are your elbow and wrist joint in alignment with your shoulder?
Are your elbow and wrist joint inside or outside the width of your shoulder?
Can you sense the strength of your alignment?

Rest.

Now for comparison, apply pressure with your fist, consciously misaligning your shoulder, elbow and wrist joint. Begin to increase your pressure by using the muscles in your arm. (10.9)

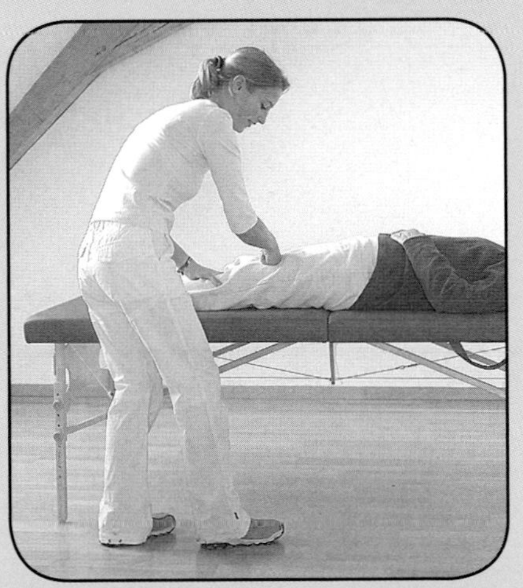

Figure 10.9

Notice how your body responds to this style of applying pressure.
Can you sense the disadvantages of misalignment?
Can you sense the consequences of using too much muscular effort?
How is your overall stability affected?
Can you breathe freely?

continued

Something to think about...

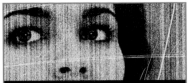

How conscious are you of your alignment when applying pressure?

____

____

____

Can you think of an activity, other than manual therapy, where you use yourself in alignment?

____

____

____

Can you think of an example where alignment generates strength and power? (Maybe you can think of an architectural example.)

____

____

____

____

____

____

____

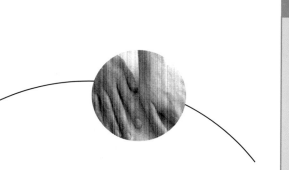

Practice tip 10.2

Does your elbow have a "mind of its own"? During your next session, notice if your elbow has the tendency to stick out, away from the alignment of your shoulder and hand. Often, out of habit, the arm is kept bent, taking the strength of alignment out of action, and replacing it with muscular effort. If you find that your arm tires quickly, check in and find out if you are unnecessarily holding your arm in flexion. If so, find a way to bring your elbow back into alignment.

Rest.

Once again, stand in a self-supported manner. Begin to apply pressure with effective alignment.

Tip Point your feet, pelvis and torso in the direction of your fist to help ensure that your body is not rotated away from your area of focus. As learned with lifting, facing your area of focus is a key point in finding effective alignment.

Once you feel comfortable, you can try applying pressure using different aspects of your hand, forearm and elbow. Use proper alignment to generate strength from your skeleton and reduce your muscular fatigue.

Partner feedback
How did having effective alignment affect the application of pressure?

_____
_____
_____

How did using misalignment affect the application of pressure?

_____
_____
_____

Which style of alignment felt better to you and your partner?

_____
_____
_____

Applying deep pressure

Many therapists believe that they must be physically strong to apply deep pressure, in addition, many clients believe that only "tall and strong" therapists can apply the "kind of pressure" they need. These beliefs are difficult to dispel and nothing could be further from the truth. With the concepts of getting close, proper alignment, self-support, counterbalance and generating power with the lower body, you have the skills required to effectively apply deep pressure.

As you have learned in Chapter 9, using your body weight to apply deep pressure is effective, but losing your sense of self-support in the process diminishes your effectiveness. As we have discussed, when you lose your self-support, you also lose your sense of control and balance. When applying deep pressure, you cannot afford to be out of control. You must maintain your control and balance, at all times, in order to insure your effectiveness, and your client's comfort.

To apply deep pressure, get close, use proper alignment and transfer your weight into your area of focus. (10.10) Depending on your intention, you can sink your weight down into the area of contact or lean your weight into it. When sinking your weight down, stand close to the area of focus, and lower yourself by bending down from your hip joints, knees and ankles. (10.11) To increase the depth, lower your stance. When leaning your weight forward, stand in close proximity and lean your weight into the area of focus by moving your entire body forward. (10.12) To increase the depth, press your feet into the ground and push forward. In both cases, bending from your hip joints, knees and ankles and counterbalancing your body will help you remain stable, strong and in control.

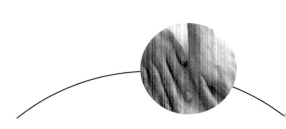

Practice tip 10.3

If you have a client who enjoys a full-body treatment with deep pressure, consider using your forearm to perform the majority of the session. The forearm provides you with the perfect tool for deep work and can cover a lot of tissue at one time. Just make sure that you keep your forearm in alignment with your shoulder and that your wrist joint stays relaxed.

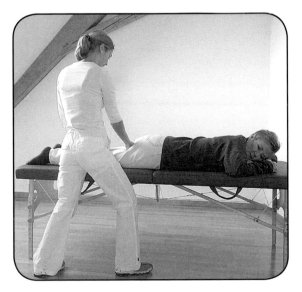

Figure 10.10

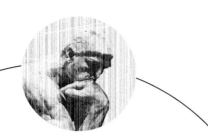

Consider this

"To more effectively deliver deep pressure with less muscular effort, you must make use of your body weight. Weight is a factor of gravity pulling down; therefore, you can only use your body weight to your advantage if you are literally over the client." [3]

Dr. Joseph E. Muscolino

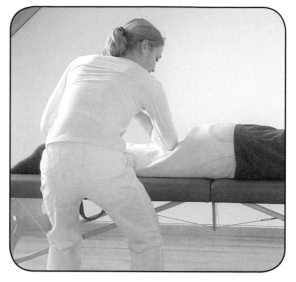

Figure 10.11

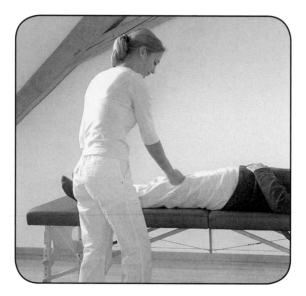

Figure 10.12

Many therapists find it helpful to lean into their table for leverage.(10.13) This is fine as long as you do not compromise your balance and control. As discussed in Chapter 9, when you find yourself in a position where all of your weight is in your hands, you have lost balance and control. Whether you lean or sink, do so by maintaining your self-support and strength of alignment.

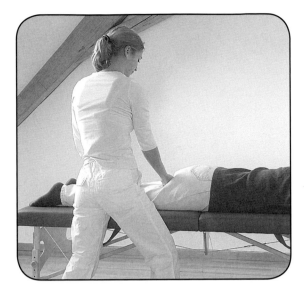

Figure 10.13

Choosing the right tool will also allow you to sink or lean your weight into an area effectively. A proximal initiation of power is more effective than a distal initiation of power.[2] For example, it is preferable to generate power from the wrist instead of the fingers, the elbow instead of the wrist, the shoulder instead of the elbow and the trunk instead of the shoulder. Thus for your application, using the elbow to applying deep pressure to larger and thick hamstrings, for example, gives a better mechanical advantage than using the fist.

The following *Partner practice* lesson gives you the opportunity to experience these concepts.

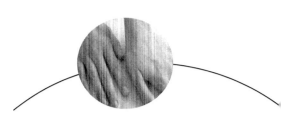

Practice tip 10.4

As a rule, it is a good idea to check in with your client, regarding depth, throughout your session. Never assume that you know, better than you client, what the right depth of pressure is, especially when applying deep pressure. Your sense of what the appropriate depth is may not be the same as your client's. Keep in verbal contact to ensure that you are always maintaining a comfortable and safe depth.

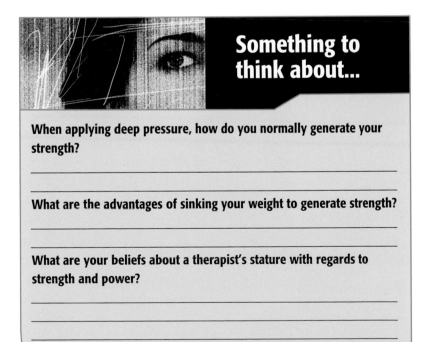

Something to think about...

When applying deep pressure, how do you normally generate your strength?

_____

_____

What are the advantages of sinking your weight to generate strength?

_____

_____

What are your beliefs about a therapist's stature with regards to strength and power?

_____

_____

_____

Applying deep pressure

Ask your partner to lie prone on your table. Choose an area on the hamstrings and stand close to it. Bending from your hip joints, knees and ankles, place your elbow on the area of focus, making sure to use proper alignment. (10.14)

*Slowly begin to **sink** your weight into your area of focus by lowering yourself down. Check in with your partner and find a comfortable depth. If your partner would like you to increase the amount of pressure, continue to lower your stance.*

Tip Keep your elbow and shoulder focused down into your pressure. Be careful not to let your shoulder rise up as you increase the pressure.

Hold the pressure for a moment and sense if you are using excessive muscular effort. If you are, reduce it by letting your body weight generate your strength. Let your hand and arm relax, keeping a self-supported stance.

Rest.

Stand as before, and apply pressure. But this time, for comparison, use excessive muscular strength, sinking all your weight onto your partner in such a way that you lose your sense of self-support. Continue to check in with your partner regarding the depth. (10.15)

Notice how your body responds to this style of applying pressure.
How does this style of applying pressure affect your shoulder and arm?
Are you able to keep your shoulder relaxed?
What happens to your breathing?
How much pressure are you able to apply?
Are you in control and balanced?

Rest.

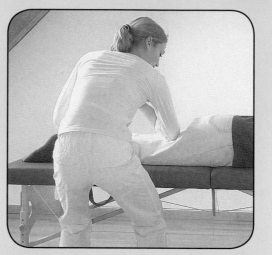

Figure 10.14

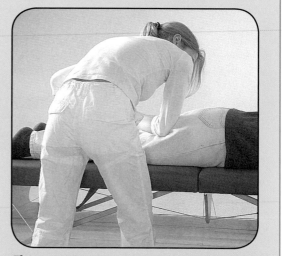

Figure 10.15

continued

Stand as before. Now return to applying pressure by using a strong alignment, sinking your weight down and maintaining your self-support. Continue to check in with your partner about the depth.

Tip With your alignment, create a line of force with your skeleton to the contact point on your partner's body.

Notice how this style feels, compared to using excessive muscular strength without self-support.
Are you able to keep your shoulder and arm more relaxed?
What is the quality of your breathing?
How much pressure are you able to apply now?
Are you in control and balanced?

Rest.

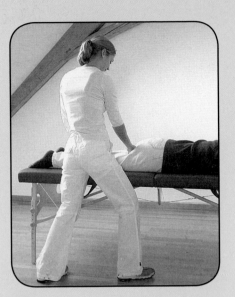

10.16

*Now, change your stance so that you are ready to **lean** your body weight forward to apply deep pressure. Stand in close proximity, in a self-supported manner. Use your fist to apply deep pressure, maintaining a strong wrist, elbow and shoulder alignment. Check in with your partner and find a comfortable depth.* (10.16)

To increase your depth, press your feet into the ground and lean your body forward. Maintain your self-support by bending from your hip joints, knees and ankles and counterbalancing your body.

Tip Pressing your feet into the ground helps to generate the power you need. Your strong skeletal alignment helps you use the strength of your bones, instead of excessive muscular effort.

Rest.

Stand as before, and apply pressure. But this time, for comparison, use excessive muscular strength, leaning all your weight forward onto your partner in such a way that you lose your self-support. Continue to check in with your partner regarding the depth. (10.17)

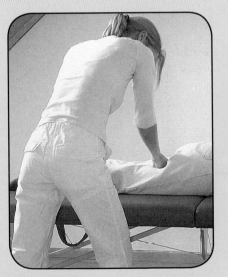

Figure 10.17

continued

Notice how your body responds to this style of applying pressure.
How does this style of applying pressure affect your shoulder and arm?
Are you able to keep your shoulder relaxed?
What happens to your breathing?
How much pressure are you able to apply?
Are you in control and balanced?

Rest.

Stand as before. Return to applying pressure by using a strong alignment, leaning your weight forward and maintaining your self-support. Continue to check in with your partner about the depth.

Notice how this style feels, compared to using excessive muscular strength without self-support.
Are you able to keep your shoulder and arm more relaxed?
What is the quality of your breathing?
How much pressure are you able to apply now?
Are you in control and balanced?

Rest.

Sinking or leaning your body weight to apply deep pressure while standing close, using good alignment and maintaining self-support allows you to use your entire body to generate strength. These concepts protect your hands from stress and utilizes the strength of your skeletal alignment and power of your lower body to generate the power needed. You can now feel confident in your ability to apply deep pressure.

Partner feedback
How did sinking and leaning your body weight affect the amount of pressure you were able to apply?

_____

_____

Did it feel as if you were able to control your pressure adequately?

_____

_____

How did using your body weight compare to using your muscular strength?

_____

_____

Breathing while applying pressure

Holding sustained pressure in one area for several seconds or minutes is common in manual therapy. When dynamic body mechanics are not used, this kind of work can often be the cause of stress and extreme fatigue. It is all too common for manual therapists, when applying sustained pressure, to slowly become stiff and static.

As you know, reducing your muscular effort will decrease stiffness and fatigue. The fewer isometric contractions your muscles hold, the more energy and vitality they will have. This is one reason why using your body weight, rather than pure muscle strength, is so important. The other important point to remember is - keep breathing.

Often therapists feel faint and quickly lose energy while applying sustained pressure. This is largely due to a shallow breathing pattern when holding still. Consciously breathing slowly and deeply when applying sustained pressure keeps your body strong and energized.

The following *Partner practice* lesson will lead you through an exploration of this concept.

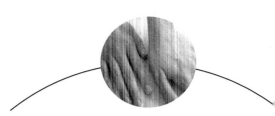

Practice tip 10.5

Conscious breathing can help reduce discomfort and increase your overall energy. If you experience discomfort while working, for example in your low back, consciously breathe into the area, taking a few minutes and focusing your breath into your low back. Breathing consciously, in general, helps to revitalize the entire body, but can also aid in comforting specific areas of stress. Your conscious breathing helps your client to remember to breathe as well!

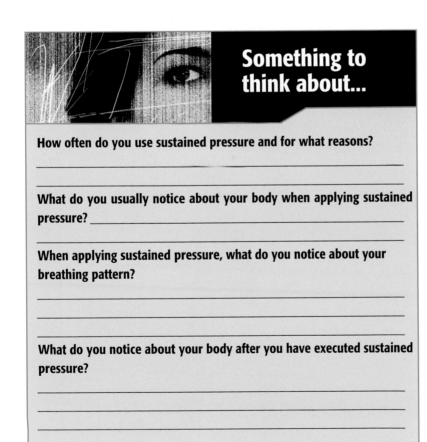

Something to think about...

How often do you use sustained pressure and for what reasons?

_____

_____

What do you usually notice about your body when applying sustained pressure? _____

_____

When applying sustained pressure, what do you notice about your breathing pattern?

_____

_____

_____

What do you notice about your body after you have executed sustained pressure?

_____

_____

_____

Breathing while applying pressure

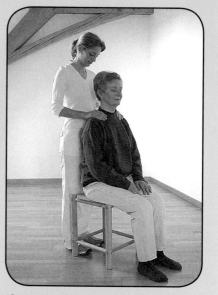

Ask your partner to sit in a chair. Stand close behind him or her. With your hands, apply pressure to your partner's shoulders. Hold the pressure for a few minutes. (10.18)

Notice how much effort you are using.
Are you tightly holding the muscles of your hands, arms and shoulders?
Are you using your body weight to apply the pressure?

Notice how you are breathing.
Are you breathing deeply or shallowly?

Figure 10.18

Rest.

Stand behind your partner, applying and holding pressure to his or her shoulders once again. Focus on using your body weight and less muscular effort in the muscles of your hands, arms and shoulders As you hold the pressure, begin to consciously breathe slowly, taking a few deep breaths. Recall the three-part breathing cycle - inhale, exhale and rest, learned in the Breathing awareness lesson in Chapter 2. (10.19)

Notice your breathing.
What parts of yourself do you feel moving as you breathe?

Continue to breathe slowly, allowing the movement of your breath to move into your entire body.

Sense the movement of your breathing in:
Your head and jaw.
Your neck and shoulders.
Your elbows and hands.
Your upper, mid and low back.
Your pelvis and hip joints.
Your legs and feet.

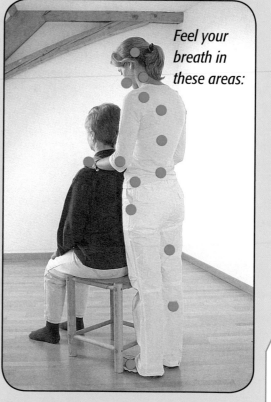

Feel your breath in these areas:

Figure 10.19

continued

As you continue to apply pressure and consciously breathe, sense how your entire body can be very alive and dynamic as you apply and hold pressure.

Rest.

Repeat this lesson using your elbow and forearm.

Consciously breathing while applying pressure is an effective way to ensure that your body stays dynamic and vital.

Partner feedback

How did consciously breathing affect your quality of touch?

_____

_____

How did your partner's body respond to your breathing?

_____

_____

What are the advantages of conscious breathing when working?

_____

_____

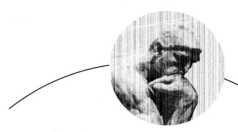

Consider this

Have you ever seen a horse sleeping while standing? The fact is, many large animals sleep when standing because their weight, when lying, presses against their rib cage, making breathing difficult. In animals like horses, giraffes and elephants, the leg joints lock automatically when standing, allowing them to breathe comfortably and remain stable, even when sleeping.[4]

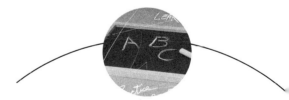

Client education tip 10.1

If a client is suffering from menstrual cramps, leading her through some simple breathing techniques may help to relieve the discomfort. Encourage her to focus her breath into her pelvis and low back, leading her through slow and deep cycles of breathing. (If needed, review Self-observation 3.3, in Chapter 2.) Breathing exercises are nice alternatives to pain medication and they don't cost a penny!

Now that you've read this chapter…

How aware are you now of how you apply pressure?

○ *almost always*
○ *sometimes*
○ *not very often*
○ *other*_____

When applying pressure, what parts of your body are you now most aware of?

○ *neck and shoulders*
○ *arms and hands*
○ *pelvis and legs*
○ *other*_____

When applying pressure, what parts of your body are you still not aware of?

○ *neck and shoulders*
○ *arms and hands*
○ *pelvis and legs*
○ *other*_____

Describe 5 concepts that make applying pressure more dynamic.

1. _____

2. _____

3. _____

4. _____

5. _____

Describe an aspect of applying pressure that is easy and comfortable.

_____

_____

Describe an aspect of applying pressure that is not yet comfortable.

_____

_____

How confident are you now applying pressure?

○ *completely*
○ *mostly*
○ *a little bit*
○ *not very*

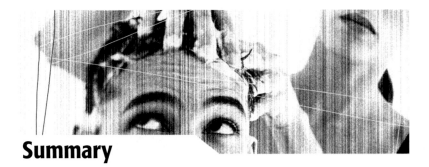

Summary

In this chapter, we have focused on applying pressure by using your body weight, effective alignment, getting close to your work and consciously breathing to help your body stay dynamic. Here is a review of the concepts learned in this chapter:

Working close is especially important when applying pressure to ensure that your body stays relaxed. **Effective alignment**, a line of support which you create by stacking your bones, enables you to use the strength of your bones, as opposed to muscular effort.

To **apply deep pressure**, get close, use proper alignment and transfer your weight into your area of focus. Depending on your intention, you can sink your weight down into the area of contact or lean your weight into it. Choosing the right tool will also allow you to sink or lean your weight into an area effectively. A proximal initiation of power is more effective than a distal initiation of power.

Consciously breathing deeply when applying sustained pressure enables your body to remain dynamic.

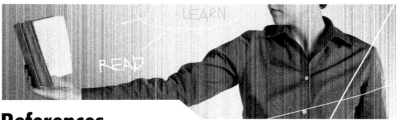

References

1.   Hall, E.T. *The Hidden Dimension.* New York: Doubleday, 1966.

2.   Muscolino, Joseph E. *Electronic Communication.* June 2003.

3.   Muscolino, Joseph E. *Electronic Communication.* June 2003.

4.   *How Does He Sleep Standing Up?* www.doesgodexist.org/MayJun96.
     6 May 2000.

A Spa Therapy

All the concepts in this book can be adapted to spa therapy, however, if you are working in a spa or considering it, this appendix will give you some extra points to keep in mind.

Water, Mineral, Herbal and Essential Oil Bath Therapies

Standing: If conditions are wet and/or slippery from, for example, essential oils, pay attention to your alignment and maintain a stable stance.

Bending: When bending down, for example, to a whirlpool or bathtub, be sure to bend from your hip joints, knees and ankles. Keep your back in a neutral position.

Lifting: When assisting a client out of a bathtub or whirlpool, get as close as possible, lift with your legs and maintain a stable stance.

Steam and Sauna

Breathing: When walking in and out of steams and/or saunas, make sure to maintain a healthy breathing pattern.

Hydration: Drink extra water. Dehydration can occur when repeatedly going from one temperature to the next.

Water Affusions

Bending: Bend from your hip joints, knees and ankles, especially when using an affusion hose for long periods of time.

Tools of the trade: Holding an affusion hose can lead to stress in your hands and arms. Keep your hands and arms as relaxed as possible, and use a variation of movements.

Affusions Under Pressure

Standing: Secure footing is imperative when using an affusion hose with a jet nozzle. Maintain your stability and alignment.

Tools of the trade: Holding an affusion hose which is under pressure requires strength in the hands and arms. Hold the hose securely, but try not to over-grip. Keep your arms close to your body to reduce muscular effort.

Showers and Steam Showers

Standing: Make sure secure footing, stability and alignment are maintained. When utilizing a Vichy shower, reach over the therapy table from a stable stance. If needed, use a step stool to increase your stability. Always reach up in alignment with the shower, avoid reaching from a rotated stance.

Body Wraps and Packs

Bending and reaching: Bend from your hip joints, knees and ankles when reaching. Whenever possible, avoid reaching across the mid–line of the table. But when you must, avoid reaching across from a rotated stance.

Facials

Sitting: When sitting for long periods of time, be sure to rest your weight on your ischial tuberosities and upper thighs, and maintain contact with your feet to the floor. Avoid working in a rotated position.

Tools of the trade: Sitting behind the client, while working with the face, can increase fatigue in the hands, arms and shoulders. Keep your shoulders in a neutral and relaxed position and work with your arms close to your body. Your fingers and thumbs should remain relaxed, yet flexible.

Exfoliation Treatments

Applying pressure: For a treatment that requires applications of pressure, such as a salt glow or body scrub, be sure to utilize your entire body, not just your shoulders, arms and hands. Whether using circular or linear movements, press your feet into the floor, transfer power from your lower body to your hands and allow your entire body to flow with your movements.

Tools of the trade: Keep your shoulders, arms and hands as relaxed as possible. Avoid over-gripping tools, such as sponges. Use a variety of movements.

B Transferring Clients

Before trying these techniques with a client, practice them with a partner. This will increase your confidence, ensuring you client's comfort and safety.

While transferring your client, stay in constant communication with him or her. Before you start, inform the client of your intentions, ensuring that there is no discomfort during or after the transfer.

If you have concerns that your client's weight and/or condition is too much for you to manage, ask someone to assist you. If assistance is not available, adapt your treatment plan so that your client can remain in their original position.

From Wheelchair to Therapy Table

Preparation: Make sure that your table is approximately the same height as the chair, and place the chair close to the table. Lock the wheels of the chair.

If possible, ask your client to sit near the edge of the chair. Place your client's feet on the floor, hip-width apart and align the ankles underneath the knees. (This ensures good skeletal alignment.) (B.1)

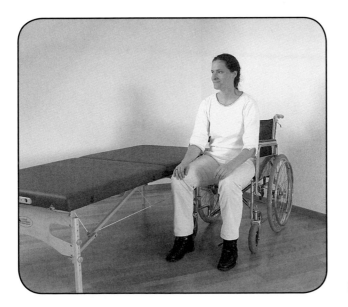

Figure B.1

Stand in a one-foot forward stance, with the forward leg in between your client's legs (this allows you to stand as close as possible). Place your arms around the client's back or shoulders and, if possible, clasp your hands together. The client's hands should be on your shoulders or wrapped around your neck.

Before starting the next sequence of movements, explain to your client what you are going to do and what he or she can do to assist you. Hold your client close to you and slowly shift your weight back so that your client's upper body leans forward. When your client's weight is approximately over his or her legs and feet, slowly straighten your legs, raising your body to bring your client's body to a standing position. (B.2, 3 & 4)

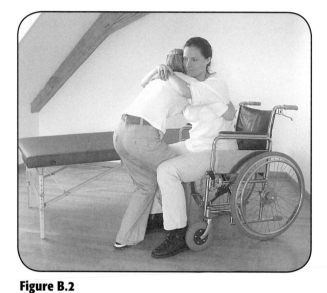

Figure B.2

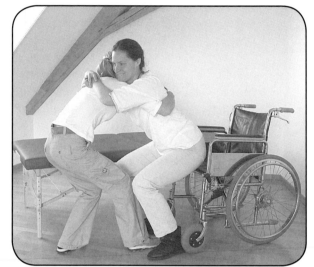

Figure B.3

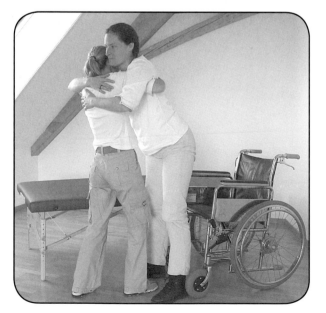

Figure B.4

Tip Keep your spine in a neutral position and your legs in alignment. Bend from your hip joints, knees and ankles. Counterbalance your weight and use the strength of your legs to move your client.

Once your client is standing, reposition yourself so that you are facing the table. Facing your table, ask and/or assist your client to turn and face you. Make sure that your client's legs have contact to the table behind him or her (this helps your client know where the table is). (B.5 & 6)

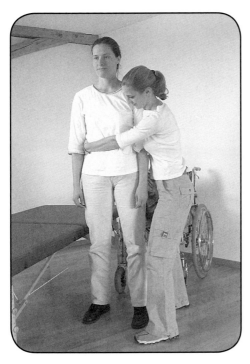

Figure B.5

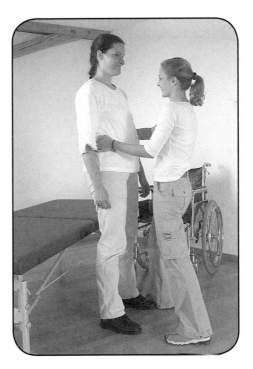

Figure B.6

From this position, you can reverse your previous movements: Stand in a one-foot forward stance, with your forward leg in between your client's legs. Place your arms around your client's back or shoulders and clasp your hands together. The client's hands should be on your shoulders or wrapped around your neck.

Before starting this next sequence of movements, as before, explain to your client what you are going to do and what he or she can do to assist you. Holding your client close, slowly shift your weight back and lower your stance. This will bring your client's upper body forward and allow him or her to bend from the hip joints, knees and ankles. When your client's pelvis is near the table, shift your weight forward and slowly lower your client to a sitting position. (B.7)

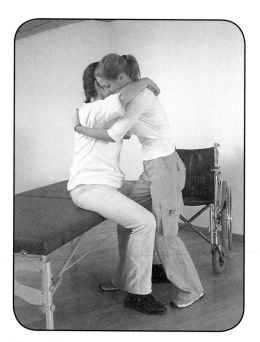

Figure B.7

From Therapy Table to Wheelchair

Preparation: Bring the chair close to the table and lock the wheels.

Begin with your client in a side-lying position. From a side-lying position, if your client is not able to come into a sitting position, bend from your hip joints, knees and ankles, with one arm, cradle the head and neck, and place the other on the upper hip. Push the hip in the direction of the feet while raising the upper body, bringing your client into a sitting position. (B.8 & 9)

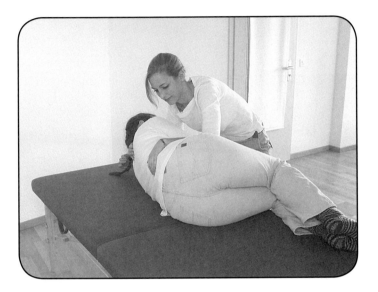

Figure B.8

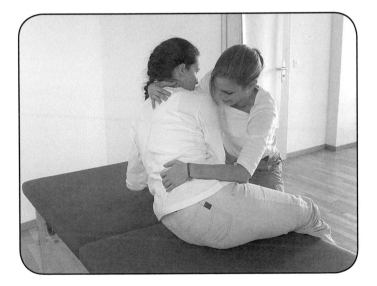

Figure B.9

If possible, ask your client to sit near the edge of the table. Place your client's feet on the floor, hip-width apart, and align the ankles underneath the knees. See B.1

Stand in a one-foot forward stance, with the forward leg in between your client's legs. (This allows you to stand as close as possible.) Place your arms around the client's back or shoulders and, if possible, clasp your hands together. The client's hands should be on your shoulders or wrapped around your neck.

Before starting this next sequence of movements, explain to your client what you are going to do and what he or she can do to assist you. Hold your client close to you and slowly shift your weight back so that your client's upper body leans forward. When your client's weight is approximately over his or her legs and feet, slowly straighten your legs, raising your body to bring your client's body to a standing position. See B.2, 3 & 4

Tip Keep your spine in a neutral position and your legs in alignment. Bend from your hip joints, knees, and ankles, counterbalance your weight, and use the strength of your legs to move your client.

Once your client is standing, reposition yourself so that you are facing the chair. Once you are facing the chair, ask and/or assist your client to turn and face you. Make sure that your client's legs have contact to the chair behind him or her. (This helps your client know where the chair is.) See B.5 & 6

From this position, you can reverse your previous movements: Stand in a one-foot forward stance with your forward leg in between your client's legs. Place your arms around your client's back or shoulders and clasp your hands together.

Before starting this next sequence of movements, as before, explain to your client what you are going to do and what he or she can do to assist you. Holding your client close, slowly shift your weight back and lower your stance. This will bring your client's upper body forward and allow him or her to bend from the hip joints, knees and ankles. When your client's pelvis is near the chair, shift your weight forward, and slowly lower your client to a sitting position. See B.7

C Other Working Surfaces

Working at a table is the main situation used in this book. However, there are several other possibilities, for example, working with your client on the floor, standing while your client is seated or getting on your table to work. Whatever your working surface, take into consideration the concepts in this book. No matter what surface you choose to work on or what position your client is in, the principles remain the same. Here are some examples of how to apply the concepts you have already learned:

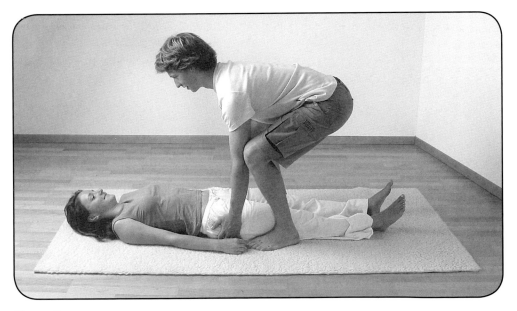

Figure C.1

- Bend from your hip joints, knees and feet.
- Counterbalance your upper body and pelvis.

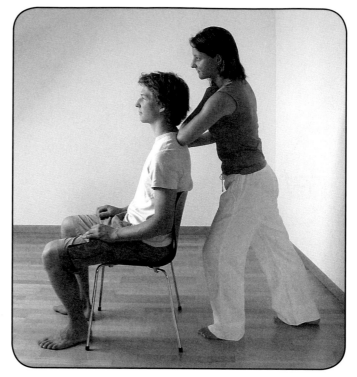

Figure C.2

- Use proper alignment.
- Sink or lean your body weight to apply deep pressure.
- Stand close and maintain self-support.

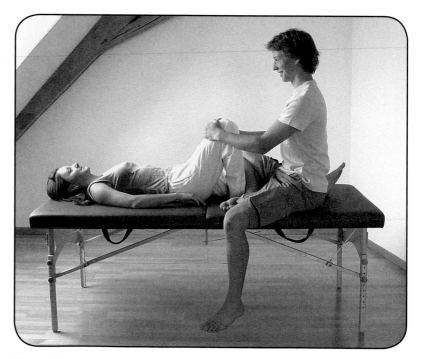

Figure C.3

- Maintain vertical alignment.
- Use the ischial tuberosities and legs as your base of support.
- Maintain proper head balance.

D Stretches

When you begin, move to the point where you feel a mild and gentle stretching. Once there, be sure to breathe and relax as you hold the stretch.

Do not bounce while holding a stretch and **never stretch to the point of pain or discomfort.**

Wrist stretches

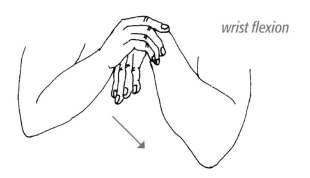

wrist flexion

wrist extension

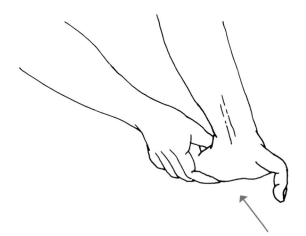

Arm, abdominal and chest stretches

lateral trunk flexors

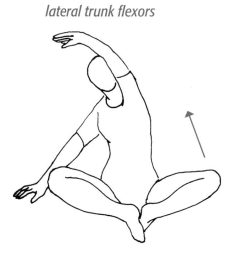

triceps

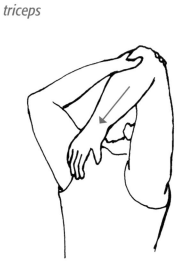

posterior shoulder

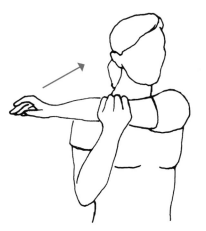

chest

chest

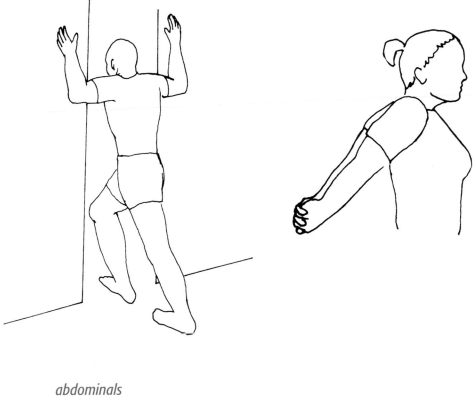

abdominals

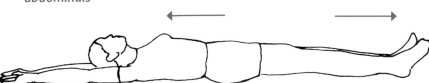

Neck and back stretches

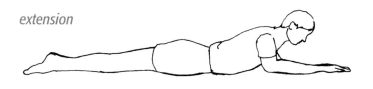

extension

flexion/extension

latissimus dorsi and shoulder

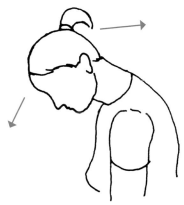

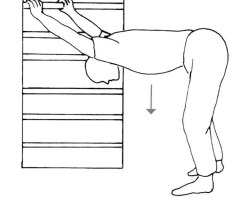

lateral side bends

back

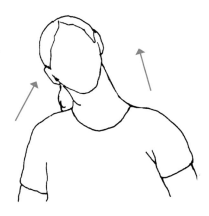

flexion/rotation

back

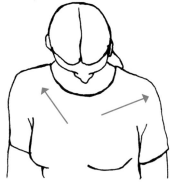

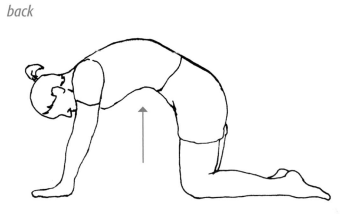

Leg and back stretches

rotation

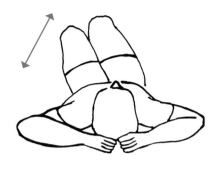

rotation

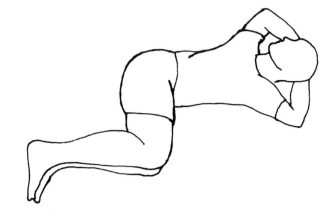

low back

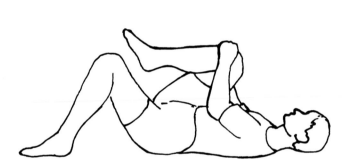

low back

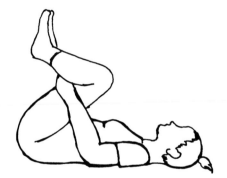

lower back and abductors

low back and hamstrings

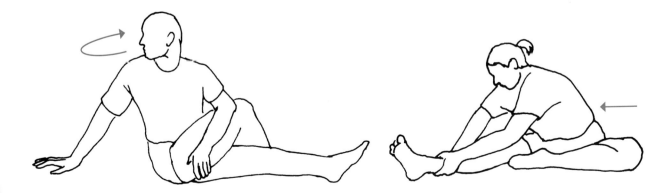

Leg stretches

quadriceps

groin

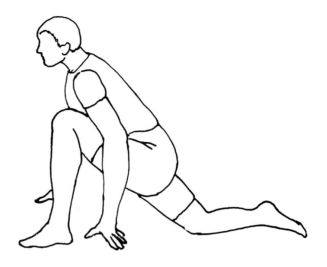

hamstrings

adductors

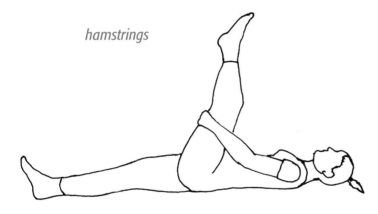

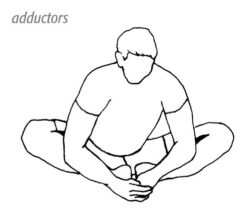

calf

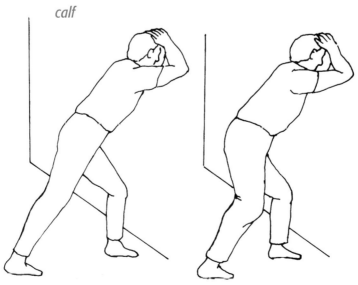

E *Troubleshooting Common Repetitive Stress Injuries*

A qualified health care practitioner should confirm and/or diagnose your symptoms, and recommend an appropriate treatment plan.

Name	What & Where	Symptoms
Median nerve compression and/or impingement "Carpal Tunnel Syndrome"	A compressed and/or impinged median nerve in the carpal tunnel of the wrist, due to repetitive use and/or sustained pressure to the heel of the hand.	Inflammation/pain in the hand/wrist, with tingling/numbness in the hand/wrist. Weakness/decreased coordination in hands and/or fingers.
Ulnar nerve compression "Guyon's Canal Syndrome"	An irritation of the ulnar nerve as it passes between the pisiform and hamate (Guyon's canal). Pressure on the ulnar nerve is usually the cause.	Pain and feeling of "pins and needles" in the ring and little finger. Decreased sensation/weakness in the hand.
Compression and/or impingement of nerves C5 to T1. "Thoracic Outlet Syndrome"	A compression and/or impingement of the brachial plexus nerves, C5-T1, in thoracic outlet (space between the first rib and clavicle). Often caused by a decrease in space due to habitual postures.	Inflammation/pain in cervical and suprascapular regions. Pain may radiate down into the triceps, inner arm, medial forearm and ulnar side of the hand.
Flexor tenosynovitis "Trigger Finger"	An inflammation of the sheath of the tendons that bend and extend the fingers and thumb. Often caused by repetitive grasping or the prolonged use of tools.	Inflammation/pain in the palm directly beneath the affected finger or thumb. Painful snapping sensation during finger movement.
DeQuervain's tenosynovitis "De Quervain's Syndrome"	An inflammation of the abductor and extensor tendon sheaths of the thumb at the radiostyloid process. Often caused from forceful gripping and sustained extension.	Inflammation/pain in the thumb and radial wrist. Pain may radiate up arm. Weakness in the thumb with adduction, abduction, extension and radial deviation.
Lateral epicondylitis "Tennis Elbow"	An inflammation of the common tendinous origin of the forearm extensor muscles, resulting from overuse/misuse.	Inflammation/pain in elbow at humeroradial joint. Pay may radiate up or down arm when at rest and/or with activity.
Rotator cuff tears "Rotator Cuff Syndrome"	A strain to any of the four rotator cuff muscles: supraspinatus, infraspinatus, teres minor and subscapularis.	Inflammation/pain/stiffness in shoulder. Pain may radiate up the neck and/or down arm when at rest and/or with activity.
Back Pain	A strain to and/or spasm in the muscles of the back, sprain to its tendons or ligaments, or slipped intervertebral discs. Often caused by bending and/or lifting with the low back.	Inflammation/pain in the associated joints, muscles, and/or intervertebral discs. Pain may radiate down the leg, up the back and/or across back and buttocks.

Self-care	Prevention	More...
Reduce inflammation and pain. Rest hand by incorporating the forearm/elbow into routine. Reduce treatment load and/or length of treatments.	Avoid hyperextension and hyper-flexion of the wrist joint. Apply compression strokes with the palmar hand. Avoid repeated use of the heel of the hand.	The Carpal Tunnel Syndrome Home Page: www.ctsplace.com
Rest activities of the hand. Incorporate the forearm/elbow into routine. Reduce treatment load and/or length of treatments.	Incorporate the use of the entire hand. For deep compression strokes, use the fist and/or forearm.	www.handsurgeon.com/guyon
Reduce inflammation and pain. Gentle stretching of the pectoralis muscles. Regular deep and slow breathing exercises.	Relax shoulders, arms & hands. Maintain upper body alignment, e.g., neck over spine. Avoid "slouched" and "jutting head " postures. Avoid repeated use of carrying straps	icongrouponline.com/health/ thoracic_outlet_syndrome
Reduce inflammation and pain. Avoid and/or modify activities causing pain.	Relax fingers and thumb, especially when grasping. When using hand tools, avoid sustained pressure of tool on the pads of the fingers.	www.indianahandcenter.com
Reduce inflammation and pain. Light cross-fiber friction at radiostyloid process. Avoid exacerbating pain.	Use the knuckles, fist and elbow for compression strokes. Avoid forceful gripping, sustained extension and radial deviation.	www.indianahandcenter.com
Reduce inflammation and pain. Trigger point work and/or light cross-fiber friction. Avoid exacerbating pain.	Avoid working with the elbow continuously flexed, and over-gripping with the hand. When using the forearm and/or elbow, keep the fingers, wrist joint and arm relaxed.	www.tennis-elbow.net
Reduce inflammation and pain. Massage and manual lymphatic drainage. Gentle movements that do not cause pain.	Keep shoulders relaxed. Avoid holding them up and/or internally rotated when working. Warm-up before starting workday.	www.jointhealing.com
Reduce inflammation and pain. Massage and gentle stretching and mobilizing.	Maintain neutral position of spine, bend and/or lift with hip joints, knees and ankles. Avoid bending and/or lifting with low back.	www.back.com

References used for Appendix E

Aland, Jeane, and King, Donna. *Deep Tissue Therapy: Theory, Technique and Application.* Garberville: Heartwood Institute, 1995.

Allard, Norman, and Barnett, Glenn. *Carpal Tunnel Syndrome. Massage and Bodywork Quarterly.* Fall 1993.

An Overview of the Research on RSI and the Effectiveness of Breaks. www.workplace.com. 15 August 2003.

Cailliet, Rene. *Hand Pain and Impairment.* Philadelphia: F.A. Davis Company, 1982.

Crouch, Tammy. *Carpal Tunnel Syndrome and Repetitive Stress Injuries.* Berkeley: Frog, Ltd. 1995.

Dixon, Marian Wolfe. *Body Mechanics and Self-Care Manual.* New Jersey: Prentice Hall, 2001.

Greene, Lauriann. *Save Your Hands: Injury Prevention for Massage Therapists.* Seattle: Infinity Press, 1995.

Lowe, Whitney. *Functional Assessment in Massage Therapy, 3rd.* Edition. Bend: OMERI, 1997.

Pascarelli, Emil, and Quilter, Deborah. *Repetitive Strain Injury.* New York: John Wiley & Sons, Inc., 1994.

Phaigh, Rich. *Tests for Thoracic Outlet Syndrome. Massage Therapy Journal.* Spring 1995.

Repetitive Strain Injuries. New York Committee for Occupational Safety and Health. www.nycosh.org.. 23 May 2003.

Tappan, Frances, and Benjamin, Patricia. *Healing Massage Techniques.* Stanford: Appleton & Lange, 1998.

Taws, Stuart. *My Hurting Hands. Massage and Bodywork Journal.* August/ September 1999.

F Bibliography

Bailey, Donna. *Track and Field.* Austin: Steck-Vaughn Co., 1991.

Bean, Constance A. *The Better Back Book.* New York: William Morrow and Company, Inc., 1989.

Biel, Andrew. *Trail Guide to the Body: How to Locate Muscles, Bones, and More!, 1st and 2nd Editions.* Boulder: Books of Discovery, 1997, 2001.

Brennan, Richard. *The Alexander Technique Workbook.* Shaftesbury: Element Books Limited, 1992.

Cailliet, Rene. *Neck and Arm Pain.* Philadelphia: F. A. Davis Company, 1981.

Cech, Donna. *Functional Movement Development Across the Life Span.* Philadelphia: W.B. Saunders Co., 1995.

Dunlap, Knight. *Habits: Their Making and Unmaking.* New York: Liveright, 1972.

Erickson, Milton H. *Life Reframing in Hypnosis.* New York: Irvington Publishers, Inc., 1985.

Falk, Dean. *Braindance.* New York: Henry Holt and Co. Inc., 1992.

Fash, Bernice. *Body Mechanics in Nursing Arts.* New York: McGraw-Hill Book Co., 1946.

Feldenkrais, Moshe. *Adventures in the Jungle of the Brain: The Case of Nora: Body Awareness as Healing Therapy.* New York: Harper & Row, 1977.

Feldenkrais, Moshe. *Awareness Through Movement: Health Exercises for Personal Growth.* New York: Harper & Row, 1972.

Feldenkrais, Moshe. *Body and Mature Behavior: A Study of Anxiety, Sex, Gravitation & Learning.* Madison: International Universities Press, 1949.

Florentino, Mary R. *A Basis for Sensorimotor Development–Normal and Abnormal.* Springfield: Charles C. Thomas, 1981.

Frost, Loraine. *Posture and Body Mechanics.* Iowa City: State University of Iowa, 1952.

Gaskin, John. *Movement.* New York: F. Watts, 1984.

Germain-Calais, Blandine, Lamotte, Andree. *Anatomy of Movement: Exercises.* Seattle: Eastland Press, 1996.

Gibson, Gary. *Pushing and Pulling.* Connecticut: Copper Beech Books, 1995.

Goldthwait, Joel E. *Essentials of Body Mechanics in Health and Disease.* Philadelphia: J. B. Lippincott, 1952.

Gray's Anatomy, 38th Edition. New York: Churchill Livingstone, 1995

Greene, Lauriann. *Save Your Hands! Injury Prevention for Massage Therapists.* Seattle: Infinity Press, 1995.

Grieve, June I. *Muscles, Nerves and Movement: Kinesiology in Daily Living, 2nd edition.* London: Blackwell Science Ltd., 1996.

Hall, Carrie M., Brody, Lori T. T*herapeutic Exercises; Moving Toward Function.* Philadelphia: Lippincott Williams & Wilkins, 1999.

Hall, Mina. *The Big Book of Sumo.* Berkeley: Stone Bridge Press, 1998.

Hall, Susan J. *Basic Biomechanics.* New York: McGraw-Hill Co., 1998.

Haller, Jeff. *Use of Self* (audio tapes) Trelleborg, Sweden: Haller, 1997.

Hoppenfield, Stanley. *Physical Examination of the Spine and Extremities.* Norwalk: Appleton & Lange, 1976.

Jacobs, Karen. *Ergonomics for Therapists.* Oxford: Butterworth-Heinemann, 1999.

Jenkins, David B. *Hollingshead's Functional Anatomy of the Limbs and Back.* Philadelphia: W. B. Saunders Co., 1991.

Johnson, Don Hanlon (Edited by). *Breath, Bone, and Gesture: Practices of Embodiment.* Berkeley: North Atlantic Books, 1995.

Juhan, Dean. *Job's Body: A Handbook for Bodywork.* Barrytown: Station Hill, 1987.

Kapandji, I. A. *The Physiology of the Joints.* New York: Church Livingstone Inc., 1987.

Kelly, Ellen D. *Teaching Posture and Body Mechanics.* New York: A.S. Barnes, 1949.

Kendall, FP, McCreary, EK. *Muscles: Testing and Function, 3rd edition.* Baltimore: Williams & Wilkins, 1983.

Leavy, Hannelore R., and Bergel, Reinhard R. *The Spa Encyclopedia: A Guide to Treatments and Their Benefits for Health and Healing.* Clifton Park: Thomson Learning Inc., 2003.

Lederman, Eyal. *Fundamentals of Manual Therapy: Physiology, Neurology and Psychology.* New York: Churchill Livingstone, Inc., 1997.

Lee, Mabel. *Fundamentals of Body Mechanics & Conditioning: An Illustrated Teaching Manual.* Philadelphia: W. B. Saunders, 1949.

Linden, Paul. *Comfort at Your Computer: Body Awareness Training for Pain-Free Computer Use.* Berkeley: North Atlantic Books, 2000.

Lippert, Herbert. *Anatomie: Text und Atlas.* Berlin: Urban & Schwarzenberg, 1976.

Malalasekera, G. P. *Encyclopedia of Buddhism.* Colombo: Government of Ceylon, 1973.

Martin, Suzanne. *Functional Movement Development Across the Life Span.* Philadelphia: W.B. Saunders Co., 1995.

Mayglothling, Rosie. *Rowing.* Wiltshire: The Crowood Press, 1990.

McMinn, R.M.H. *Color Atlas of Human Anatomy.* Chicago: Year Book Medical Publishers, 1985.

Mitchell, Stewart. *The Complete Illustrated Guide to Massage.* Great Britain: Element Books Limited, 1997.

Mumford, Susan. *Healing Massage: A Practical Guide to Relaxation and Well-Being.* New York: Penguin Putman Inc., 1997.

Peterson, Roger T. *Field Guide to Animal Tracks (Peterson Field Guides).* Oxfordshire: Houghton Mifflin Co., 1998.

Platzer, Werner. *Color Atlas and Textbook of Human Anatomy, Volume 1: Locomotor System, 3rd edition.* New York: Thieme Inc., 1986.

Reynolds, Edward. *The Evolution of the Human Pelvis in Relation to the Mechanics of the Erect Posture.* Cambridge: The Museum, 1931.

Roaf, Robert. *Posture.* New York: Academic Press, 1977.

Roberts, Tristan, D. M. *Understanding Balance: The Mechanics of Posture and Locomotion.* New York: Chapman & Hall, 1995.

Rolf, Ida P. *Rolfing: Reestablishing the Natural Alignment and Structural Integration of the Human Body.* Rochester: Healing Arts Press, 1989.

Rolf, Ida. *Rolfing and Physical Reality.* Rochester: Healing Arts Press, 1990.

Rolf, Ida. *Rolfing: Integration of Human Structures.* New York: Harper Row, 1977.

Salvo, Susan G. *Massage Therapy: Principles and Practice.* Philadelphia: W.B. Saunders, 1999.

Schumacher, John A. *Human Posture: The Nature of Inquiry.* New York: State University of New York Press, 1989.

Sechi, Davide. *Massage Basics.* New York: Sterling Publishing Co., 1998.

Shafarman, Steven. *Awareness Heals: The Feldenkrais Method for Dynamic Health.* Massachusetts: Addison-Wesley Publishing Co., 1997.

Sivananda Yoga Vedanta Center. *Yoga Mind and Body.* New York: Dorling Kindersley, 1996.

Staub, Frank. *Mountain Goats.* Minneapolis: Lerner Publications Co., 1994.

Tappan, Frances M., Benjamin, Patricia J. *Tappan's Handbook of Healing Massage Techniques, 3rd edition.* Stamford: Appleton & Lange, 1998.

Thompson, Clem W. *Manual of Structural Kinesiology, 11th edition.* St. Louis: Times Mirror/ Mosby College, 1989.

Thompson, Diana L. *Hands Heal: Communication, Documentation, and Insurance Billing for Manual Therapists, 2nd Edition.* Baltimore: Lippincott Williams & Wilkins, 2002.

Todd, Mabel E. *The Thinking Body.* Brooklyn: Dance Horizons, 1979.

Tortora, Gerald. *Principles of Human Anatomy, 4th edition.* New York: Harper & Row, 1986.

Tozeren, Aydin. *Human Body Dynamics: Classical Mechanics and Human Movement.* New York: Springer-Verlag, 1999.

Tyldesley, Barbara. *Muscles, Nerves and Movement: Kinesiology in Daily Living, 2nd edition.* London: Blackwell Science Ltd., 1996.

Vogel, Steven. *Cats' Paws and Catapults: Mechanical Worlds of Nature and People.* New York: W. W. Norton & Co., 1998.

Wilson, Frank. The Hand: How Its Use Shapes the Brain, Language, and Human Culture. New York: Vintage Books, 1998.

Zacharkow, Dennis. *Posture: Sitting, Standing, Chair Design and Exercise.* Springfield: Charles C. Thomas, 1988.

Zacharkow, Dennis. *The Healthy Low Back.* Springfield: Charles C. Thomas, 1984.

World Wide Web Sources

Back and Neck Care Guide. McKinley Health Center, University of Illinois. February 8, 2000 Retrieved: March 3, 2000 from the World Wide Web: http://www.uiuc.edu.departments/
mckinley/health-info/fitness/back

Die Entwicklung im 1. Lebensjahr

Retrieved: April 3, 2000 from the
World Wide Web: http://www.home.wtal.de/uerhage/
babyentwicklung.htm

Southeastern Hand Center. Surgery of the Hand and Upper Extremity. Jack L. Greider.

Retrieved: April 17, 2000 from the World Wide Web: http://www.handsurgery.com

Study: Human Ancestors had Knuckle-Walking Characteristics. March 22, 2000. Associated Press. Retrieved: April 17, 2000 from the World Wide Web: http://www.cnn.com/2000/nature/03/22/
knuckle.walkers.ap

Index